D1503446

THE MEDICAL WORD FINDER:

A REVERSE MEDICAL DICTIONARY

Betty Hamilton and Barbara Guidos

Neal-Schuman Publishers, Inc.
New York   London

Published by Neal-Schuman Publishers, Inc.
23 Leonard Street
New York, NY 10013

Library of Congress Cataloging-in-Publication Data

Hamilton, Betty.
    The medical word finder.

    1. Medicine—Dictionaries.   2. Synonyms.   I. Guidos,
Barbara.   II. Title.   [DNLM: 1. Nomenclature.
W 15 H217m]
R121 .H232 1987   610' .3'21   86-28462
ISBN 1-55570-011-X

CONTENTS

PREFACE

The language of any highly specialized profession can be extremely intimidating to those not intimately acquainted with the field. This is especially true in the medical profession, whose language is so obscure that it seems as though only "insiders" can possibly understand it. Those not well-versed in medical terminology know how time-consuming it is to find medical words in medical dictionaries where entries often are defined by terms that are themselves so technical that one can spend a good deal of time perusing cross-references or consulting other sources.

The Medical Word Finder: A Reverse Medical Dictionary is a tool for identifying technical medical terminology from common words and phrases. While it is not intended to replace a medical dictionary, it is a useful supplement for persons with extensive medical background as well as those with little medical knowledge. It is designed to aid researchers, writers, editors, students, and lay persons to locate quickly medical terms without having to consult numerous references and primary sources or go back and forth through a medical dictionary. It will also serve as a quick reference for healthcare professionals and those in allied fields.

The 10,000 terms in *The Medical Word Finder* originate from working lists compiled by the authors over several years from major medical references as well as hundreds of other sources. They cover a broad range, from commonly used terms and phrases such as "baldness," "dizzyness," "thirst," "water pill," "face lift," and "bone surgery," to more specified terms such as "dysentery," "cornea rupture," "cauterization," and "apoplexy." Entries include synonyms and closely related terminology, and, where appropriate, comprehensive lists of commonly used prefixes and suffixes that form the fundamentals of medical etymology. For example, the prefix "dys-" will be found under abnormal, bad, and difficult. Under the entry "condition" you will find the suffixes "-asia, -esis, -iasis, -ism, -osis, -sis," along with "derangement, disease, disorder," and "dysfunction."

Many medical terms are now part of our everyday language, yet many people have only a vague notion of their meanings, the proper contexts in which they are used, and their variety of nuances. *The Medical Word Finder* will help readers bring these words into focus. For example, if you know that osteoporosis refers to some kind of bone disease, you can look in *The Medical Word Finder* under the headings related to "bone" to find osteoporosis listed under bone loss.

As in most translations, whether from one language to another or—within the same language—from idiomatic usage to professional argot, there are relatively few "pure" synonyms. The medical field is no exception. However, words commonly used to describe physical states, sensations, or medical procedures are often "umbrella" terms which in the medical profession cover a variety of specific diseases, symptoms, and treatments. The terms and expressions in *The Medical Word Finder* extend the scope of common terms to include a plethora of meanings.

The phrase "chest pain," for example, may refer to many conditions; under this entry, you will find such words as myocardial infarction, angina, hiatus hernia, hyperventilation, pericarditis, pulmonary embolus. Each refers to a distinct condition but shares a common symptom. Under the entry "mix" is listed amalgamate, coalesce, compound, cross-breed, cross-fertilize, homogenize, hybrid, interbreed, synthesize. These terms have connotative differences and may be used in several medical contexts.

The Medical Word Finder lists not only single words but extended phrases that further delineate terms. Under the heading "abdomen," you will also find "abdomen, air in; abdomen, contents removed; abdomen fissure; abdomen incision; abdomen opening; abdomen puncture," etc.

Also provided in this reference are extensive lists of medications which in common parlance may be referred to by a single, generic term. For instance, the entry "antihistamines" lists 36 varieties (acrivastine, chlorpheniramine, hydroxyzine, meclizine, etc.); "cancer therapy" lists more than 100 kinds of cancer drugs.

Among the many other types of entries included in *The Medical Word Finder* are parts of the body, with lists of their specific anatomical structures; lists of amino acids, enzymes, and other chemical substances in the body; extensive lists of disease entities and disease-causing agents such as viruses, bacteria, and fungi;

nearly 100 terms under "pain in," from pain in the abdomen to pain in the vessels; more than 100 types of surgical and diagnostic instruments; and a comprehensive list of phobias.

The Medical Word Finder also contains entries for unusual or aberrant physical and psychological phenomena, such as abnormal grin (risus sardonicus), Hottentot bustle (steatopygia), and involuntary sound (aboiement), as well as commonplace words— gag, fear of lightning, twitching—which many people may not realize actually have a variety of medical terms.

The Medical Word Finder follows the letter-by-letter style of alphabetizing up to the first punctuation mark. For example, "leg, wasting of" is followed by "legal" and "leg calf." The order of words under the entries is usually alphabetical, although the most commonly used synonyms may be listed first, and listings for anatomical structures may follow the classic head-to-toe order.

Alphabetized Listing
of Words and Phrases

A

abdomen: abdomino-, celio-, -ventral,
ventri-, ventro-, abdominal cavity,
bladder, colon, gallbladder,
genitals, intestinal tract, kidneys,
large intestine, liver, pancreas,
peritoneum, small intestine,
splanchna, spleen, stomach, viscera
See also specific organs

abdomen, air in: pneumoperitoneum

abdomen, contents removed:
eventration, evisceration,
exenteration

abdomen, dropsy: ascites

abdomen, pus in: pyocelia,
pyoperitoneum

abdomen disease: celiopathy

abdomen distension: meteorism,
tympanites, tympany

abdomen examination: abdominoscopy,
celioscopy, laparoscopy, ventroscopy

abdomen excision: celiectomy,
laparectomy, laparohysterectomy,
laparosalpingo-oophorectomy

abdomen fissure: celoschisis,
schistocelia

abdomen hernia: enterocele,
epigastrocele, eventration,
splanchnocele

abdomen incision: celioenterotomy,
celiogastrotomy, celiomyomotomy,
celiotomy, laparotomy, ventrotomy

abdomen inflammation: celiomyositis,
celitis, laparomyitis, peritonitis

abdomen opening: colostomy,
cystostomy, ectocolostomy,
enterostomy, ileostomy, ostomy

abdomen pain: abdominalgia,
celiomyalgia, splanchnodynia

abdomen prolapse: panoptosis,
splanchnoptosis, visceroptosis

abdomen puncture: abdominocentesis,
amniocentesis, celiocentesis,
celioparacentesis, paracentesis,
peritocentesis

abdomen regions: hypochrondriac,
epigastric, lumbar, umbilical,
inguinal, hypogastric

abdomen sounds: borborygmus

abdomen surgery: laparogastrostomy,
laparotomy, ventrofixation
See also specific organs

abdomen suturing: celiorrhaphy

abdomen tumor: carcinoma,
celiothioma, mesothelioma
See also specific organ tumors

abnormal: all-, dys-, mal-, para-,
aberrant, abortion, anomaly,
deformity, deviant, dyscrasia,
heteronomous, malformation,
mutant, perversion, polymeria,
psychopathic

abortifacient: carboprost, dinoprost,
dinoprostone

abortion: embryoctony, embryotocia

abortion, induced: abactus venter

abortion, sign of: Tarnier's

abortion fever: brucellosis

abortion producing: aborticide,
abortifacient

abortion therapy: dydrogesterone,
medroxyprogesterone

about: ambi-, peri-

above: ep-, epi-, hyper-, super-,
supra-

abscess: apostasis, apostem, empyema,
fester, ulcer, ulceration

abscess, urine in: urapostema

absence of: a-, an-, non-

absorption: assimilation, chondrolysis,
digestion, dissolved, imbibition,
osmosis

absorption inducing: sorbefacient

absorption through skin: endermic,
transdermal

abuse: addiction, molestation, rape

acceleration: auxo-

accessory parts: adnexa, annexa,
appendage, collateral, concomitant

accidental: adventitious

accommodation: adjustment, focusing

according to: cata-
accumulation: accretion
acetone in blood, excessive:
    acetonemia
acetone in urine: aceturia
acetone poisoning: dimethylketone
    toxicity, propanone toxicity
acetylcholine effects: cholinergic
acetylcholine receptor blockage:
    anticholinergic
ache: pain, spasm, throb
Achilles tendon: tendo calcaneus
Achilles tendon incision: achillotomy
Achilles tendon inflammation:
    achillobursitis, Albert's disease
Achilles tendon pain: achillodynia
Achilles tendon suturing:
    achillorrhaphy
acid: -ate, acescent, acidum, LSD
acid accumulation: acidemia, acidosis
acid head: LSD user
acid in stomach, excess: chlorhydria
acid in urine: aciduria
acidity, deficient: anacidity
acidity reducer: antacid
acidosis: Butler-Albright syndrome,
    Lightwood's syndrome, renal
    hyperchloremia
acid production: oxyntic
acid-secreting cell: parietal
acid tide: aciduria
acnelike: acneform, acneiform
acne therapy: dapsone, isotretinoin,
    resorcinol, tretinoin
acquired: adventitious, inherited
acrid: acid, caustic, pungent
across: trans-
act against: counteract
acted on: -ate
action: -asis, -ergy
action potential: electrical charge,
    facilitation
actions, unconscious: automatism,
    telergy
active: sthenic
activity, excessive: tumultus

activity, lack of: anergy
Adam's apple: larynx, pomum adami
adaptation: accommodation, coping,
    facultative
added: adjunct, appendage
addiction: alcohol abuse, dependence,
    drug abuse, substance abuse
addition to: ad-
adenoid: pharyngeal tonsil
adenoids removed: adenoidectomy
adhesion: accretion, conglutination,
    synechia
adhesion causing: desmoplastic
adhesion surgery: adhesiotomy,
    synechotomy, synechtenterotomy
adjustment: acclimation,
    accommodation, adaptation,
    coping, facultative
adolescent medicine: ephebiatrics,
    ephebology
adrenal cortex hormones: aldosterone,
    androgens, androstenedione,
    dehydroepiandrosterone, estrogens,
    glucocorticoids, mineralocorticoids
adrenal cortex tumors: adenomas,
    aldosteronoma
adrenal gland: adreno-
    See also gland, hormone
adrenal gland, increased activity:
    adrenarche
adrenal gland, inhibitory agent:
    adrenostatic
adrenal gland, produced by:
    adrenogenous
adrenal gland activity: -adrenia
adrenal gland diseases: Achard-Thiers
    syndrome, adrenalopathy,
    adrenopathy, aldosteronism, Conn's
    disease, Cushing's syndrome,
    Schmidt's syndrome, Waterhouse-
    Friderichsen syndrome
adrenal gland enlargement:
    adrenomegaly
adrenal gland inflammation:
    adrenalitis, adrenitis, epinephritis
adrenal gland insufficiency: Addison's
    disease, hypoadrenalism

adrenal gland removal: adrenalectomy
adrenal gland stimulation:
   adrenokinetic, adrenotropic
adrenal gland supression: adrenopause
adrenal gland toxin: adrenotoxin
adrenal gland tumors: paraganglioma,
   pheochromocytoma
Adrenalin: *See* epinephrine
adrenal nonfunctioning: anadrenalism
adrenocortical suppressants:
   aminoglutethimide, trilostane
adrenocorticoids: amcinonide,
   beclomethasone, betamethasone,
   ciprocinonide, clobetasol,
   clobutasone, clocortolone, cortisone,
   desonide, desoximetasone,
   desoxycorticosterone,
   dexamethasone, diflorasone,
   diflucortolone, fludrocortisone,
   flumethasone, flumoxonide,
   fluocinolone, fluocinonide,
   fluorometholone, flurandrenolide,
   halcinonide, hydrocortisone,
   methylprednisolone, naflocort,
   paramethasone, prednisolone,
   prednisone, procinonide,
   timobesone, tipredane,
   triamcinolone
adsorbent: activated charcoal, kaolin
affective disorders: bipolar,
   cyclothymic, depression, dysthymia,
   hypomanic, manic, mood
   disturbance, neurotic personality
affinity: trop-, -trophism, tropo-,
   -tropy
after: meta-, post-
afterbirth: placenta, secundines
afterbrain: pons and cerebellum
aftereffect: residual
again: an-, ana-, pali-, palin-, re-
against: ant-, anti-, cata-, contra-,
   contraindication
age: achievement, adolescent,
   anatomic, bone, childhood,
   chronologic, developmental,
   emotional, functional, geriatric,
   gestational, menarche, mental,
   physiologic, puberty

aggravate: exacerbate
aggregated: acervuline
aging: senescence
aging, premature: progeria
aging, study of: geriatrics,
   gerontology
aging specialist: geriatrician,
   gerontologist
agitated: corybantism, restive,
   tumultus
air: aer-, aero-, physo-, pneum-,
   pneuma-, pneumato-, pneumatic
air, absence of: anaerobic
air, fear of: aerophobia
air, impurity measurement instrument:
   cacaerometer
air, lack of: dyspnea
air, provide: ventilation
air hunger: dyspnea
air in abdomen: pneumoperitoneum
air in cerebral ventricles:
   pneumoventricle
air in pleural cavity: pneumatothorax,
   pneumothorax
air in spinal canal: pneumatorachis
airless: anaerobic
airlike: aeriform, gaseous
air passages: alveolus, bronchiole,
   bronchus, mouth, nose, trachea
air removal: exsufflation
air sac: aerocele, alveolus
air swallowing: aerophagia
air therapy: aerohydrotherapy,
   aerotherapy, aerothermotherapy
airtight: hermetic
albumin in bile: albuminocholia
albumin in blood: albuminemia
albumin in blood, absence:
   analbuminemia
albumin in blood, decreased:
   hypoalbuminemia
albumin in blood, increased:
   hyperalbuminemia
albumin in sputum: albuminoptysis
albumin in urine, excessive:
   albuminaturia, albuminorrhea,
   albuminuria, proteinuria

albumin-like: albuminoid
albumin producing: albuminogenous
alcohol: ethanol
alcohol deterrent: disulfiram
alcohol in blood: alcoholemia
alcohol in urine: alcoholuria
alcoholism: alcoholomania,
  alcoholophilia, delirium tremens,
  dipsomania, enomania,
  intoxication, Korsakoff's psychosis,
  methomania, oinomania,
  posiomania
alcohol withdrawal therapy:
  clorazepate
aldosterone antagonist: canrenoate,
  canrenone, dicirenone, mexrenoate,
  prorenoate, spironolactone
aldosterone secretion, excessive:
  aldosteronism, hyperaldosteronism
Aleppo boil: cutaneous leishmaniasis
algae, study of: algology, phycology
alienation: anomie
alimentary canal: digestive tract
alimentation: mastication, swallowing,
  digestion, absorption, assimilation;
  nourishment
alive: breathing, extant, viable
alkali in urine: alkalinuria, alkaluria
alkaline accumulation: alkalosis
alkaline depletion: acidosis, alkalipenia
alkalizer: sodium bicarbonate,
  tromethamine
alkylating agents: busulfan,
  chlorambucil, cisplatin,
  cyclophosphamide, dacarbazine,
  lomustine, melphalan
all: pan-, pant-, panto-
allantois: allanto-
allergic: atopic
allergic reaction: anaphylactic
  hypersensitivity, anaphylactic
  shock, anaphylaxis, cell-mediated
  hypersensitivity, cytotoxic
  hypersensitivity, hyperergy,
  hypersensitivity, hypoergy,
  immune complex hypersensitivity,
  pathergy

allergic to oneself: autoimmune
allergy, study of: allergology
allergy causing: allergen
allergy therapy: antihistamines,
  brompheniramine,
  chlorpheniramine, cromolyn,
  cyproheptadine,
  dexbrompheniramine,
  diphenhydramine, minocromil,
  nivimedone, phenyltoloxamine,
  pirquinozol, promethazine,
  proxicromil, tiacrilast, tixanox
alleviate: palliate
alloy: amalgam
almond-shaped: amygdalo-,
  amygdala, amygdaloid
aloneness, fear of: autophobia,
  eremophobia, monophobia
along: sym-
alternate: all-
alveolus: alveolo-
alveolus inflammation: alveolitis
ameba, destructive to: amebicide
ameba in urine: ameburia
amebalike: amebiform, ameboid
amebicides: carbasone, chloroquine,
  iodoquinol, paromomycin
amenorrhea therapy: bromocryptine
  mesylate
amines, excess in urine: aminosuria
amino acid defect: aminoacidopathy
amino acids: alanine, arginine,
  aspargine, citrulline, cysteine,
  cystine, glutamic acid, glycine,
  hydroxyglutamic acid,
  hydroxyproline, norleucine, proline,
  serine, tyramine, tyrosine
amino acids, essential: isoleucine,
  leucine, lysine, methionine,
  phenylalanine, threonine,
  tryptophan, valine; histidine,
  arginine
amino acids, pathologic production:
  aminosis
amino acids in blood, excessive:
  aminoacidemia,
  hyperaminoacidemia

amino acids in urine, excessive:
aminoaciduria
amino-fatty acids: aminolipid
aminoglycosides: amikacin,
gentamycin, kanamycin,
neomycin, netilmicin,
streptomycin, tobramycin
ammonia: ammoni-
ammonia excretion: ammonirrhea
ammonia in blood, excessive:
ammonemia, ammoniemia
ammonia in urine, excessive:
ammoniuria
amnion: amnio-
amnion rupture: amniorrhexis
amniotic fluid, excessive: hydramnios,
polyhydramnios
amniotic fluid, loss of: amnioclepsis,
amniorrhea
amniotic fluid deficiency: hypamnios,
oligohydramnios
amniotic fluid test: amniocentesis
amniotic sac examination:
amniography
amplification: enlargement, expansion,
magnification
ampule inflammation: ampullitis
amputation: apocope, cineplastics,
kineplasty, loxotomy, truncate
amylase in urine, excessive:
amylasuria
analgesic therapy: acetaminophen,
acupressure, acupuncture,
aminobenzoate, anidoxime,
anilopam, antipyrine, aspirin,
bicifadine, bromadoline,
buprenorphine, butorphanol,
carbiphene, ciprefadol, ciramadol,
clonixin, codeine, dezocine,
diflunisal, dimefadane,
doxpicomine, drinidene,
ethoxazene, fenoprofen,
floctafenine, flupirtine, fluradoline,
hydrocodone, hydromorphone,
ibuprofen, imipramine, ketazocine,
ketorfanol, letimide, levorphanol,
mefenamic acid, meperidine,
methadone, methopholine,
methotrimeprazine, metkephamid,

mimbane, molinazone, morphine,
nabitan, nalbuphine, namoxyrate,
nantradol, naproxen, nexeridine,
octazamide, opium, oxycodone,
pentazocine, picenadol, prodilidine,
profadol, propiram, propoxyphene,
pyrroliphene, salicylamide,
sufentanil, tazadolene, tilidine,
tramadol, veradoline, volazocine,
zenazocine, zomepirac
anal skin sore: anal fissure, anal fistula
anal wink: anal sphincter contraction
analytic methods: Addis count, assay,
chromatography, electron
microscopy, electrophoresis,
microscopy, spectrophotometry
See also diagnostic aids, tests
anaphylaxis preventive:
ananaphylaxis, antianaphylaxis,
desensitization
anatomical snuffbox: tabatiere
anatomique
anatomy: applied, comparative,
descriptive, gross, microscopic,
morbid, pathologic, surface,
surgical
anatomy, pathologic:
anatomicopathologic
anatomy specialist: anatomist
ancestor: progenitor
ancestry: -clinous
anchor-shaped: ancyroid
androgens: fluoxymesterone,
mesterolone, methyltestosterone,
nandrolone, oxandrolone,
oxymetholone, testosterone
androgens, excess in female:
androgenization
androgen stimulating: andromimetic
anemia: drepanocytemia,
erythroblastosis fetalis, pernicious,
sickle cell, thalassemia, toxanemia
anemia preventive: antianemic
anemia therapy: cyanocobalamin,
ferrous sulfate, fluoxymesterone,
hydroxocobalamin, leucovorin

anesthesia: block, electroanesthesia, general, local, pudendal, regional, saddle block, toponarcosis
anesthesia, conduction: nerve block
anesthesia, science of: anesthesiology
anesthesia specialist: anesthesiologist, anesthetist
anesthetics: aliflurane, benoxinate, benzocaine, bupivacaine, butacaine, butamben, chloroform, chloroprocaine, cocaine, cyclomethycaine, cyclopropane, dexivavaine, diamocaine, dibucaine, diperodon, diphenhydramine, dyclonine, enflurane, ether, etidocaine, etoxadrol, euprocin, fluroxene, halothane, hexylcaine, isobucaine, isobutamben, isoflurane, ketamine, lidocaine, mepivacaine, meprylcaine, methohexital, methoxyflurane, midazolam, minaxolone, nitrous oxide, norflurane, obtundent, oxethazaine, phenacaine, phencyclidine, pramoxine, prilocaine, procaine, propanidid, proparacaine, propoxycaine, pyrrocaine, risocaine, rodocaine, roflurane, sevoflurane, teflurane, tetracaine, thiamylal, thiopental, tiletamine
aneurysm excision: aneurysmectomy
aneurysm incision: aneurysmotomy
aneurysm repair: aneurysmoplasty
aneurysm suturing: aneurysmorrhaphy
anger, violent: furor
angina-like: anginiform
angina pectoris: stenocardia
angina pectoris, fear of: angiophobia
angle: bend, elbow, flexure, knee
angles, measurement of: goniometry
animal-like: zooid
animal research: callisection, vivisection

animals, abnormal love for: zoomania, zoophilism
animals, fear of: zoophobia
animal skins, fear of: doraphobia
animal toxin: zootoxin
ankle: talo-
ankle, formed by: fibula, tibia, talus
ankle fracture: Wagstaffe's fracture
ankle jerk: Achilles reflex
ankle joint: articulation, diarthrosis, ginglymus, hinge, talocrual, talotibiofibular
ankle pain: talalgia, tarsalgia
ankle surgery: tarsectomy
antacid: algedrate, almadrate, aluminum hydroxide, dihydroxyaluminum, magaldrate, magnesium carbonate, polyethadene, silodrate
antagonistic: histoincompatible, incompatible
ant bite irritation: formiciasis
anterior: proso-
anteroposterior: directio-
anthelmintics: albendazole, anthelmycin, bromoxanide, butonate, cambendazole, clioxanide, closantel, cyclobendazole, dribendazole, etibendazole, fenbendazole, gentian violet, hexylresorcinol, mebendazole, metronidazole, niclosamide, nitrodan, oxamniquine, oxfendazole, oxibendazole, parbendazole, piperazine, praziquantel, pyrantel pamoate, pyrvinium, rafoxanide, tetracloroethylene, thiabendazole, ticarbodine, tioxidazole, vincofos, zilantel
antianginal drugs: acebutolol, amlodipine, amyl nitrate, atenolol, bepridil, betaxolol, cinepazet, diltiazem, metoprolol, nadolol, nicardipine, nifedipine, nitroglycerin, oxprenolol, pindolol, propranolol, timolol, tosifen, verapamil

antiarrhythmia drugs: acebutolol, atenolol, bretylium, deslanoside, digitalis, digitoxin, digoxin, diltiazem, disopyramide, edrophonium, lidocaine, methoxamine, metoprolol, nadolol, oxprenolol, phenytoin, procainamide, propranolol, quinidine, timolol, tocainide, verapamil

antibiotics: amphotericin, bacitracin, chloramphenicol, chlortetracycline, clindamycin, colistin, erythromycin, flucytosine, griseofulvin, ketoconazole, lincomycin, miconazole, novobiocin, nystatin, oxytetracycline, paulomycin, polymyxin, rifampin, spectinomycin, spectromycin, streptomycin, tetracycline, troleandomycin, vancomycin, viomycin
See also aminoglycosides, cephalosporins, penicillins

antibodies: agglutinins, antitoxin, bacteriolysins, opsonins, precipitin

antibody formation: immunogen, immunostimulant

antibody-inducing substance: anahormone, antigen

antibody in serum: antiserum

anticholinergics: atropine, benapryzine, benzilonium, clidinium, dexetimide, elantrine, elucaine, eucatropine, ethylbenztropine, homatropine, hyoscyamine, metoquizine, oxyphencyclimine, parapenzolate, proglumide, promazine, propantheline, tiquinamide, tofenacin, toquizine, triampyzine, tropicamide

anticoagulants: acenocoumarol, ancrod, anisindione, heparin, phenindine, phenprocoumon, warfarin

anticonvulsant drugs: acetazolamide, albutoin, amobarbital, atolide, carbamazepine, cinromide, citenamide, clonazepam, clorazepate, cyheptamide, diazepam, dimethadione, divalproex, eterobarb, ethosuximide, ethotoin, fluzinamide, lamotrigine, lorazepam, mephenytoin, mephobarbital, metharbital, methetoin, methsuximide, nabazenil, nafimidone, nitrazepam, paraldehyde, paramethadione, pentobarbital, phenacemide, phenobarbital, phensuximide, phenytoin, primidone, ropizine, secobarbital, stiripentol, sulthiame, trimethadione, valproic acid, zonisamide

antidepressants: *See* depression therapy

antidiabetic agents: *See* diabetes therapy

antidiuretic hormone: vasopressin

antidiuretics: argipressin, desmopressin, lypressin, vasopressin
See also diuretic drugs

antidotes: acetylcysteine, activated charcoal, amyl nitrite, atropine, cholestyramine, colestipol, deferoxamine mesylate, dimercaprol, edrophonium, glucagon, hyoscyamine, leucovorin, mannitol, menadiol, neostigmine, nitroprusside, penicillamine, physostigmine, phytonadione, prazosin, protamine, pyridostigmine, pyridoxine

antiemetics: benzquinamide, buclizine, chlorpromazine, cyclizine, dimenhydrinate, diphenidol, diphenyhydramine, domperidone, dronabinol, flumeridone, haloperidol, hydroxyzine, meclizine, metoclopromide, metopimazine, perphenazine, prochlorperazine,

promethazine, scopolamine,
thiethylperazine, triflupromazine,
trimethobenzamide

antifungals: acrisorcin, ambruticin,
amphotericin B, azaconazole,
bifonazole, candicidin, carbol-
fuchsin, chlordantoin, ciclopirox,
clioquinol, clotrimazole, econazole,
enilconazole, filipin, flucytosine,
gentian violet, griseofulvin,
haloprogin, hamycin,
hydroxystilbamidine, itraconazole,
ketoconazole, miconazole,
natamycin, nystatin, orconazole,
parconazole, partricin, potassium
iodide, pyrrolnitrin, rutamycin,
sinefungin, thiram, tioconazole,
tolnaftate, triacetin, triafungin,
undecylenic acid, viridofulvin,
zinoconazole

antihemorrhagics: aminocaproic acid,
carboprost, desmopressin,
dinoprostone, epinephrine,
oxytocin, phytonadione, tranxemic
acid, vasopressin

antihistamines: acrivastine,
antazoline, azatadine,
bromdiphenhydramine,
brompheniramine, carbinoxamine,
chlorcyclizine, chlorpheniramine,
cinnarizine, clemastine, cyclizine,
cyproheptadine,
dexbrompheniramine,
dexchlorpheniramine,
dimenhydrinate,
diphenylhydramine,
diphenylpyraline, dorastine,
doxylamine, hydroxyzine,
levocabastine, loratadine,
meclizine, phenindamine,
phenyltoloxamine, promethazine,
pyrabrom, pyrilamine,
pyrrobutamine, rotoxamine,
tazifylline, terfenadine,
trimeprazine, tripelennamine,
triprolidine

antihypertensives: acebutolol,
alseroxylon, althiazide, amiquinsin,
atenolol, atiprosin,
bendroflumethiazide, benzthiazide,
bethanidine, bevantolol, bucindolol,
bupicomide, captopril,
chlorothiazide, chlorthalidone,
clonidine, cyclothiazide,
deserpidine, diazoxide, doxazosin,
enalapril, flordipine, furosemide,
guanabenz, guanethidine,
guanoxabenz, hydralazine,
hydrochlorothiazide,
hydroflumethiazide, indapamide,
indoramin, labetalol,
mecamylamine, methyclothiazide,
methyldopa, metolazone,
metoprolol, minoxidil, nadolol,
nifedipine, nitrendipine, ofornine,
oxprenolol, pargyline, pazoxide,
pindolol, polythiazide, prazosin,
propranolol, quinethazone,
rauwolfia serpentina, reserpine,
saralasin, spironolactone, timolol,
tinabinol, tiodazosin, triamterene,
trichlormethiazide, trimazosin,
trimethaphan
See also diuretics

anti-infection: phylaxis

anti-inflammatory agents: aspirin,
bufexamac, fenoprofen, ibuprofen,
indomethacin, meclofenamate,
naproxen, sulindac, tolmetin
See also adrenocorticoids

antinauseants: buclizine, cyclizine,
naboctate

antineoplastic agents: *See* cancer
therapy

antiseptic: bactericide, cadexomer
iodine, chlorocresol, disinfectant,
germicide, isomerol, mecetronium
ethylsulfate

antiviral agents: *See* virus therapy

anus: archo-, fundament

anus, artificial: enteroproctia

anus, imperforate: ankyloproctia,
aproctia, proctatresia

anus inflammation: architis,
periproctitis, perirectitis, proctitis
anus specialist: proctologist
anus surgery: Amussat's operation,
anoplasty, fissurectomy,
hemorrhoidectomy
anvil-shaped: incudiform, incus
anxiety: anomie, panic, pavor
anxiety disorder: obsessive-compulsive,
panic, phobias, post-traumatic
stress
anxiety treatment: alprazolam,
amalgam, anxiolytic, bromazepam,
chlordiazepoxide, chlormezanone,
clorazepate, diazepam, halazepam,
hydroxyzine, ketazolam,
lorazepam, meprobamate,
oxazepam, prazepam, tranquilizers
aorta calculus: aortolith
aorta dilation: aortectasia
aorta disease: aneurysm, aortopathy,
atherosclerosis
aorta examination: aortography
aorta excision: aortectomy
aorta incision: aortotomy
aorta inflammation: aortitis,
endaortitis, mesaortitis,
periaortitis
aorta narrowing: aortarctia,
aortostenosis
aorta pain: aortalgia
aorta rupture: aortoclasia
aorta suturing: aortorrhaphy
aorta wall hardening: aortosclerosis
aorta wall softening: aortomalacia
apart: di-
apathetic: anomie, phlegmatic, torpent
apathy: torpor
apelike: pithecoid
aperture: opening
aponeurosis incision: aponeurotomy
aponeurosis inflammation:
aponeurositis
aponeurosis suturing:
aponeurorrhaphy
apophysis inflammation: apophysitis

apoplexy: brain hemorrhage,
cerebrovascular accident, ictus,
stroke
apoplexy, after: postictal
apparent: patent, phanic
appearance: spectro-
appearance, old at young age: progeria
appearance, youthful at advanced age:
agerasia
appendage: adnexa, appendix, tag
appendix calculus: appendicolithiasis
appendix dilation: appendicectasis
appendix diseases: appendicism,
appendicopathy
appendix inflammation: appendicitis,
endoappendicitis, periappendicitis,
perityphlitis
appendix pain: appendalgia
appendix removal: appendectomy,
appendicectomy
appendix surgery: appendicolysis,
appendicostomy
appetite, abnormal: acoria,
allotriogeustia, allotriophagy,
bulimia, geophagia, parorexia, pica,
polyphagia, xenorexia
See also eating disorders, food,
hunger
appetite, lack of: anepithymia,
anorexia
appetite, reduced: dysorexia, fastidium
appetite control in brain: appestat
appetite stimulant: aperitive,
orexigenic
appetite suppressants: benzphetamine,
diethylpropion, fenfluramine,
mazindol, phendimetrazine,
phenmetrazine, phentermine,
phenylpropanolamine
apprehension: anxiety, fear
approach: aditus
appropriate: ortho-
arachnoid membrane: arachn-,
arachno-
arachnoid membrane inflammation:
arachnitis, arachnoiditis,
basiarachnitis

arch: fornix
arc-welders disease: siderosis
arising within: endogenous
arm: brachi-, brachio-, humerus,
    radius, ulna, carpus; appendage,
    brachium, upper extremity
    See also digit, extremity, hand, leg,
    limb
arm, abnormal: brachiocyrtosis,
    perobrachius
arm, long: macrobrachia
arm, small: microbrachia
arm, upper: brachium
arm bend: cubitus, elbow
arm fracture: Barton's, Colles',
    Galeazzi, Monteggia's, Moore's,
    Skillern's, Smith's
arm muscles: anconeus, biceps,
    brachialis, brachioradialis,
    extensors, flexors, pronator teres,
    triceps
arm pain: brachialgia
armpit: ala, axilla, axillary fossa,
    maschale
armpit muscle: latissimus dorsi
arms, absence: abrachia,
    abrachiocephalia, acephalobrachia
arms, paralysis: Erb's palsy
arms and legs: acral, brachiocrural,
    extremities
arms and legs, absence: amelia
around: ambi-, amphi-, circum-, peri-
arrowlike: sagittal
arsenic eating: arsenicophagy
arsenic poisoning: arseniasis,
    arsenicism
arsenic test: Marsh's
arsenic therapy: arsenotherapy
art: techno-
arteries, major: aorta, axillary,
    brachial, carotid, celiac, coronary,
    femoral, iliac, intercostal, peroneal,
    popliteal, radial, renal, subclavian,
    superior mesenteric, tibial, ulnar
artery: arteri-, arterio-, arteriole
    See also blood vessel, vein

artery, terminal: telangion
artery calcification: arteriostenosis
artery calculus: arteriolith
artery degeneration: arteriasis
artery dilation: arteriectasis
artery disease: arteriomyomatosis,
    arterionecrosis, arteriopathy
artery examination: arteriography
artery excision: arteriectomy
artery hardening: arteriolosclerosis,
    arteriosclerosis, atherosclerosis
artery incision: arteriotomy
artery inflammation: arteriolitis,
    arteritis, endarteritis, mesarteritis,
    periarteritis, polyarteritis,
    thromboarteritis
artery narrowing: arteriarctia,
    arteriostenosis
artery pain: arteralgra
artery rupture: arteriorrhexis
artery softening: arteriomalacia
artery spasm: arteriospasm
artery surgery: artioplasty,
    arteriosympathectomy
artery suture: arteriorrhaphy
artery wall degeneration: atheroma
artery wall tension: vasotonia
arthritis: chondrocalcinosis,
    degenerative, enteropathic, gouty,
    hypertrophic, infectious,
    inflammatory, juvenile rheumatoid,
    Lyme, noninflammatory,
    polyarticular, pseudogout,
    rheumatoid, Still's disease,
    suppurative, traumatic
arthritis in extremities: acroarthritis
arthritis preventive: antiarthritic
arthritis therapy: allopurinol, aspirin,
    auranofin, aurothioglucose,
    azathioprine, benoxaprofen,
    chloroquine, choline salicylate,
    colchicine, diclofenac, diflunisal,
    fenoprofen, gold sodium
    thiomalate, hydroxychloroquine,
    ibuprofen, indomethacin,
    ketoprofen, meclofenamate,
    methotrexate, naproxen,
    oxyphenbutazone, penicillamine,

phenylbutazone, piroxicam,
probenecid, salsalate, steroids,
sulfinpyrazone, sulindac, tolmetin
articulation: amphiarthrosis,
amphidiarthrosis, joint, junctura,
pronunciation
artificial body part: prosthesis
artificial kidney: hemodialysis
artificial opening: ostomy
artificial respiration: resuscitation,
transamination
asbestos-causing diseases: asbestosis,
mesothelioma
asbestos-like: asbestiform
Ascaris infection: ascariasis
asheslike: cineraceous
aspect: norma
aspirin: acetylsalicylic acid
assisting: ancillary
asthma complication: acetonasthma
asthma preventive: antasthmatic,
antiasthmatic
asthma therapy: albuterol, atropine,
beclomethasone, bitolterol,
bronchodilators, cromolyn,
dexamethasone, dyphylline,
ephedrine, epinephrine, flunisolide,
isoetharine, isoproterenol,
metaproterenol, terbutaline,
theophylline, triamcinolone
astigmatism, corrected: anastigmatic
astringent: anastaltic, apocrustic,
astriction, stypsis
asymmetric: deviation, skewed
ataxia-like: atactiform
athlete's foot: dermatophytosis,
ringworm
athlete's heart: cardiac hypertrophy
atmospheric pressure injury:
aerodontalgia, aerosinusitis,
aerotitis, barodontalgia,
barosinusitis, barotitis, barotrauma
atomizer: hydroconion
atrium: atrio-
atrophy: emaciation, macies
atrophy, skin: anetoderma, wasting

atrophy preventive: antatrophic
attach: affix, anastomosis, insert
attachment: anchorage, appendage,
fixation
attack: epilepsy, ictus, illness onset,
seizure
attention deficit: dysbulia
attitudes, conflicting: ambivalence
auscultation, cardiac: tracheophonesia
auscultation sounds: bronchophony,
bruissement, bruit, click,
crepitation, egophony,
hyperphonesis, hypophonesis,
murmur, pectoriloquy,
pectorophony, rale, rhonchus,
souffle, tracheophony, tragophony,
vesicular murmur
automatism: vigilambulism
autonomic nervous system:
parasympathetic, sympathetic,
vegetative
autopsy: necropsy, obduction,
postmortem
aviation medicine: aeromedicine
awareness: consciousness
away from: ab-, abs-, di-, ex-, abient,
distad, distal, efferent
awkward: sinistrous
axilla: ala, axillary fossa, maschale
axillary: alar
axillary gland inflammation:
maschaladenitis
axilla tumor: maschaloncus
axis: ax-, axio-, axon-
axon, absent: anaxon

B

baby: child, infant, neonate, newborn
baby, evaluation at birth: Apgar score
baby, unborn: abortus, conceptus,
embryo, fetus, zygote
bacilli, caused by: bacilligenic,
bacillogenic
bacilli, fear of: bacillophobia

bacilli in blood: bacillemia
bacilli in urine: bacilluria
bacilli producing: bacilliculture,
    bacilligenic, bacilliparous,
    bacillogenic
bacillus-like: bacilliform
back: dorsi-, dorso-, lumbo-, noto-,
    opisth-, opistho-, re-, un-, dorsal,
    dorsalis, dorsum, notal, posterior,
    tergum
back, between ribs: dorsointercostal
back, middle of: dorsomesial
back, toward: dorsiduct
backbone: rachis, spinal column,
    vertebral column
backed up: constipated
backflow: reflux, regurgitation
back muscles: latissimus dorsi,
    oliocostals, sacrospinalis, serratus,
    teres, trapezius
back pain: dorsalgia, dorsodynia,
    lumbago, lumbodynia, notalgia,
    rachialgia
backward: an-, ana-, retro-, dorsad,
    dorsal
backward displacement:
    retrodeviation, retrodisplacement,
    retroversion
backward flexion: dorsiflexion
bacteremia: Waterhouse-Friderichsen
    syndrome
bacteria: bacilli-, bacter-, bacterio-,
    Acinetobacter, Actinomyces,
    Bacillus, Bacteroides, Bartonella,
    Bordetella, Borrelia, Brucella,
    Campylobacter, Chlamydia,
    Clostridium, coccus,
    Corynebacterium, Diplococcus,
    Enterobacter, Enterococcus,
    Escherichia, Francisella,
    Fusobacterium, germ, Hemophilus,
    Klebsiella, Lactobacillus,
    Legionella, Leptospira, Listeria,
    microbe, microorganism,
    Mycobacterium, Neisseria,
    Nocardia, Pasteurella,
    Propionibacterium, Proteus,
    Pseudomonas, Rickettsia,
    Salmonella, Sarcina, Serratia,

Shigella, spirochete,
    Staphylococcus, Streptococcus,
    Treponema, Veillonella, Vibrio,
    Yersinia
    See also fungus, virus
bacteria, science of: bacteriology,
    microbiology
bacteria, treatment with:
    bacteriotherapy
bacteria action: fermentation
bacteria destruction: antibacterial,
    bactericidal, bactericidin,
    bacteriocidin, bacterioclasis,
    bacteriolysant, bacteriolysin,
    bacteriolysis, bacteriophage,
    disinfectant, microbicide
bacteria diseases: actinomycetoma,
    actinomycosis, anthrax,
    bacteremia, bacteriosis,
    bartonellosis, bejel, botulism,
    brucellosis, cholera, diphtheria,
    endocarditis, enteritis, epiglottitis,
    frambesia, gonorrhea,
    Legionnaire's, leprosy, leptospirosis,
    listeriosis, lymphogranuloma
    venereum, melioidosis, meningitis,
    meningococcemia, nocardiosis,
    pasteurellosis, pertussis, pinta,
    plague, pneumonia, psittacosis, Q
    fever, relapsing fever,
    rickettsialpox, Rocky Mountain
    spotted fever, salmonellosis,
    septicemia, shigellosis, syphilis,
    tetanus, toxic shock syndrome,
    trachoma, tuberculosis, tularemia,
    typhoid fever, typhus, yaws,
    yersiniosis
bacteria fixation: bacteriopexy
bacteria in blood: bacteremia
bacteria inhibition: bacteriostasis
bacteria in semen: bacteriospermia
bacteria in urine: bacteriuria, coliuria
bacterial changing: bacteriotropic,
    opsonic
bacterialike: bacteriform, bacterioid
bacterial vaccine: bacterin

bacteria producing: bacteriogenic
bad: cac-, caci-, caco-, dys-, mal-,
    mis-
bad breath: bromopnea, halitosis,
    ozostomia
bad odor: cacosmia
bad taste: cacogeusia
Bagdad boil: leischmaniasis
bag of waters: amniotic fluid sac
bag-shaped: sac, sacciform
baker legs: genu valgum
balance: equilibrium, scale, symmetry
balance, poor: disequilibrium,
    dizzyness, vertigo
balance test: electronystagmography
bald: acomia, alopecia, calvities,
    decalvant, glabrate, phalacrosis,
    pseudopelade, Quinquaud's disease
Balkan grippe: Q fever
ball-shaped: globoid, globular,
    spheroid
band: desm-, desmo-, bundle,
    ligament, tract, zona
bandage: abdominal, accipiter, Ace,
    Barton's, Baynton's, binder,
    butterfly, capeline, cast, compress,
    cravat, Desault's, dressing, elastic,
    Esmarch's, figure-of-eight,
    Fricke's, galea, Galen's,
    Garretson's, gauntlet, gauze,
    Gibney, habena, Hamilton's,
    hammock, ligature, many-tailed,
    Martin's, pad, plaster, pressure,
    Ribble's, Richet's, roller, Sayre's,
    scultetus, sling, spica, spiral,
    splenium, splint, strapping,
    suspensory, T, Theden's,
    tourniquet, triangular, truss,
    Velpeau's, Y
bandy-leg: genu varum
barber's itch: sycosis vulgaris, tinea
    barbae
barbiturates: amobarbital,
    aprobarbital, butabarbital,
    mephobarbital, metharbital,
    pentobarbital, phenobarbital,
    secobarbital, talbutal

barren: impotent, infecund, infertile,
    sterile
barrier: claustrum
Bartholin's glands inflammation:
    bartholinitis
bartonellosis: Carrion's disease, Oroya
    fever, verruga peruana
base: basi-, basio-, baso-, alkali,
    fundus
basketball heels: talon noir
bath, sweat: sauna, sudatorium,
    turkish
bathe: ablution, balneum, douche,
    flush, irrigate, lavage, sponge,
    swab
bathing, excessive: ablutomania
baths, as treatment: balneotherapy
baths, science of: balneology
battered child: child abuse
beadlike: moniliform
beaklike: coracoid, rostral
beard: barba
beard, excessive growth: pogoniasis
beard, first: pappus
beard in women: pogoniasis
bear young: childbirth, fecundity,
    fertile, parturition
beat: palpitation, pulsatile, pulsation,
    pulse, throb
beating: quassation
bedbug: Acanthia lectularia, Cimex
    lectularius
bedclothes, pluck at: carphology,
    floccillation
bed-shaped: clinoid
bedside care: clinical medicine,
    nursing
bedsore: decubitus ulcer
bed treatment: clinotherapy
bedwetting: enuresis
bees, fear of: apiphobia, melissophobia
beetle disease: scarabiasis
before: ante-, antero-, fore-, pre-,
    pro-, anterior, previa
beginning: arch-, arche-, archi-
behavior, study of: psychiatry,
    psychology, sociology

behavior disorder: antisocial
personality disorder, dysergasia,
sociopathic personality
behavior therapy: *See* psychologic
therapies
behind: post-, retro-
belch: eructation, ructus
believe wrongly: delusion
belladonna alkaloids: atropine,
belladonna, hyoscyamine,
scopolamine
belly: abdomen, stomach
belly ache: colic, gastralgia
belly breathing: diaphragmatic
breathing
belly-button: navel, umbilicus
belly-shaped: venter
belong to: -an, -ian
below: hypo-, infra-, sub-
bend: clino-, curvi-, arcuation,
curvature, curve, flex, geniculum
bend backward: dorsiflexion,
dorsoflexion, recurve, retroflexion
bend downward: deorsumduction
bend forward: antecurvature,
anteflect, anteflexion
bending: anfractuous, elastic, pliable
bend inward: inflexion, introflexion
bends: aeremia, aeroembolism,
aeropathy, caisson disease,
decompression sickness, dysbarism,
nitrogen narcosis
beneath: hypo-, infra-, sub-, inferior
bent: anchylo-, ancylo-, ankylo-,
geniculate
bent inward: varus
bent outward: valgus
berry-shaped: bacciform
beryllium poisoning: berylliosis
beside: para-
beta-lactam antibiotics:
cephalosporins, penicillins
between: inter-
beyond: extra-, hyper-, para-, super-,
trans-, ultra-
bicuspid valve: mitral valve

big: meg-, megal-, megalo-
bile: bili-, chol-, chole-, cholia-, cholo-,
fel, gall
See also gallbladder
bile, abnormal secretion: acholia,
oligocholia, paracholia
bile, absent: acholia
bile, absent in urine: acholuria
bile, albumin in: albuminocholia
bile, diluted: hydrocholeresis
bile, excessive: biliousness, hypercholia,
polycholia
bile, thick: pachycholia
bile calculus: choledocholithiasis,
cholelith, cholelithiasis, chololith
bile calculus crushing:
cholecystolithotripsy,
choledocholithotripsy,
cholelithotripsy
bile calculus removal:
choledocholithotomy, cholelithotomy
bile disease: dyscholia, jaundice
bile duct: choledochus
bile duct dilation: choledochectasia
bile duct disease: cholepathia
bile duct examination:
cholangiography, choledochography
bile duct excision: choledochectomy
bile duct incision: cholangiotomy,
choledochotomy, cysticotomy
bile duct inflammation: angiocholitis,
cholangiolitis, cholangitis,
choledochitis, periangiocholitis,
pericholangitis
bile duct pain: cholecystalgia, colic
bile duct repair: choledochoplasty
bile duct surgery:
cholangioenterostomy,
cholangiogastrostomy,
cholangiostomy,
choledochoduodenostomy,
choledochoenterostomy,
choledochostomy
bile duct suturing: choledochorrhaphy
bile flow inducer: cholagogue
bile formation: biligenesis, cholepoiesis

bile in blood: cholemia
bile in peritoneum: choleperitoneum
bile in spinal fluid: bilirachia
bile in urine: choleuria, choluria
bile in vomitus: cholemesis
bile pigments: bilicyanin, biliflavin,
    bilifuscin, biliprasin, bilirubin,
    biliverdin
bile secretion: choleresis
bile secretion, excessive: cholorrhea
bile secretion stimulant: chloretic
bile secretion stoppage: cholestasis
bile tract: common bile duct,
    duodenum, gallbladder, liver,
    pancreas
bilirubin in blood, excessive:
    bilirubinemia, hyperbilirubinemia
bilirubin in urine: biliurea
binge eating: bulimia
biological clock: circadian rhythm
biologicals: antigen, antitoxin, serum,
    toxoids, vaccine
biology specialist: biologist
birds, fear of: ornithophobia
birth: accouchement, childbirth,
    confinement, delivery, labor, natal,
    parturition, tocus
birth, before: antenatal, prenatal
birth, present at: congenital
birth canal: uterus and vagina
birth control: oligogenics
    See also contraceptives
birth control pill: oral contraceptive
birth defect: anomaly, congenital,
    protal
    See also congenital diseases,
    genetics, hereditary diseases
birth injury: brachial palsy, Dejerine-
    Klumpke syndrome, fracture,
    intracranial hemorrhage
birthmark: angioma, mole, nevus,
    port-wine stain
birth rate: natality, natimortality
birth rate, reduced: oligonatality
births, multiple: polytocous, twining
bisexual: amphigenetic,
    hermaphrodite, intersexual,
    pseudohermaphrodite

bite: balanced, cross, edge-to-edge,
    laceration, lesion, occlusion, open,
    over, underhung, wound
bite, poor: malocclusion
bite oneself: autophagia
biting, tongue or cheek: odaxesmus
biting edge: occlusal
bitter: picr-, picro-, acrid, amaroidal,
    picrogeusia
black: melano-, nigri-, nigro-,
    melaniferous
black and blue: contusion, ecchymosis,
    livedo, livid, suggillation
black bile: humor
Black Death: bubonic plague
black eye: hematoma
black fever: kala-azar
blackhead: comedo
black lung: anthracosis,
    pneumoconiosis
blackout: unconsciousness
black pigment: melanin, nigrites
blacks, fear of: negrophobia
black tongue: glossophytia,
    melanoglossia, nigrities linguae
bladder: cyst-, cysti-, cystido-, cysto-,
    vesico-, cystic, vesica
bladder, in front of: prevesical
bladder, near: paravesical
bladder absent: acystia
bladder base: trigone
bladder bleeding: cystistaxis,
    cystorrhagia
bladder calculus: cystolithiasis
bladder discharge: cystorrhea,
    cystoschisis
bladder disorder: acystinervia
bladder enlarged: cystauxe,
    megabladder, megalocystis
bladder examination: aerocystoscopy,
    cystography, cystoradiography,
    cystoscopy, cystourethroscopy,
    cystovesiculography,
    pneumocystography
bladder excision: cystectomy
bladder fixation: cystopexy

bladder hernia: cystocele,
  cystoepiplocele, vesicocele
bladder incision: cystotomy,
  cystotrachelotomy, vesicotomy
bladder inflammation: colicystitis,
  cystitis, cystopyelitis,
  cystopyelonephritis, cystoureteritis,
  endocystitis, epicystitis,
  paracystitis, pericystitis,
  radiocystitis
bladder neck inflammation:
  trachelocystitis
bladder pain: aplalgia, cystalgia,
  cystodynia
bladder paralysis: cystoplegia
bladder prolapse: cystocele, cystoptosis
bladder-shaped: vesical
bladder spasm: cystospasm
bladder surgery: autocystoplasty,
  cystectasy, cystoelytroplasty,
  cystolithectomy, cystoplasty,
  cystorectostomy, cystostomy,
  lithocystotomy, lithotomy,
  proctocystoplasty, proctocystotomy,
  vesicostomy
bladder suturing: cystorrhaphy,
  ventrocystorrhaphy
bladder tumor: cystoscirrhus,
  cystosarcoma
bleaching: dealbation
bleeder: hemophiliac
bleeding: epistaxis, hematemesis,
  hematuria, hemoptysis,
  hemorrhage, menorrhagia,
  menstruation, metrorrhagia
bleeding, excessive: -rhage, -rhagia,
  hemorrhage
bleeding, stopping: acutorsion,
  angiopressure, angiostrophy,
  anthemorrhagic, antihemorrhagic,
  arteriostrepsis, arterioversion,
  electrohemostasis, hemostasis,
  tourniquet
bleeding disorder: hemophilia,
  thrombocytopenia,
  thrombocytopenic purpura, von
  Willebrand's disease

blemish: birthmark, blotch, comedo,
  macula, mole, nevus, spot, wart
blind colon: appendix vermiformis
blindness: typhlo-, ablepsia, amaurosis,
  Braille, flash blindness,
  hemeralopia, object blindness,
  typhlosis
  See also color blind, eye, vision
blindness, night: nyctalopia,
  nyctotyphlosis
blindness, partial: aknephascopia,
  amblyopia, flittering scotoma,
  fortification spectrum,
  hemiamaurosis, hemiamblyopia,
  hemianopia, hemiopia, meropia,
  obcecation, quadrantanopsia,
  scintillating scotoma, teichopsia
blindness, study of: typhlology
blindness, twilight: aknephascopia
blind spot: optic disk, optic papilla,
  scotoma, scotomization
blink continuously: blepharism
blister: vesico-, bleb, bulla, phlyctena,
  phlyctenula, phlyctenule,
  pompholyx, pomphus, pustule,
  sudamen, vesication, vesicle
blistering agent: Spanish fly, vesicant
blisterlike: phlyctenoid, physaliform
bloating: dilation, distension, swollen,
  turgid
blockage: constipation, ileus,
  impaction, obstruction, obturation,
  occlusion, oppilation, stenosis
blocking agents: alpha-adrenergic,
  antiadrenergic, anticholinergic,
  beta-adrenergic, calcium channel,
  cholinergic, ganglionic, histamine
  H receptors, neuromuscular
blood: hem-, hema-, hemat-, hemato-,
  hemo-, sangui-, sanguino-, humor,
  plasma, sanguine, sanguis, serum
blood, albumin in: albuminemia
blood, albumin in, excess:
  hyperalbuminemia
blood, albumin in, low:
  hypalbuminenia, hypoalbuminemia

blood, blue: cyanemia
blood, dark: melanemia
blood, excess: hyperemia
blood, fear of: hematophobia,
  hemophobia
blood, full of: hematose
blood, high acid content: acidemia
blood, increased pH: alkalemia
blood, menstrual, retained:
  hematocolpometra, hematocolpos,
  hematosalpinx, hematotrachelos
blood, oozing of: angiostaxis,
  hemophilia
blood, pus in: pyotoxinemia
blood, reduced volume: oligemia
blood, science of: hematology
blood, thick: pachyemia, pachyhemia
blood, tinged: sanguinolent
blood, urates in: uratemia
blood, vomiting: hematemesis
blood accumulation: hematocele,
  hematocolpos
blood alcohol: alcoholemia
blood amino acids, excessive:
  aminoacidemia
blood bicarbonate, low: acarbia
blood calculus: hemolith
blood capillaries, in kidney: glomeruli
blood carbon dioxide, reduced:
  acapnia, hypocapnia
blood cell destruction: hemocytolysis,
  hemolysin, hemolysis
blood cell development:
  hematogenesis, hematopoiesis,
  hemocytogenesis
blood cell fragment: schistocyte
blood cells: basophil, corpuscle,
  erythrocyte, granulocyte,
  hemocyte, leukocyte, lymphocyte,
  monocyte, platelet, reticulocyte,
  thrombocyte
  See also red blood cells, white blood
  cells
blood cells, decreased: aplastic anemia,
  hematocytopenia, pancytopenia
blood cells, measurement: hematocrit,
  sedimentation rate

blood cells, removed: cytapheresis,
  erythropheresis, leukapheresis,
  lymphapheresis,
  lymphoplasmapheresis,
  plasmapheresis,
  thrombocytapheresis
blood cells, study of: hematology,
  hemocytology
blood cell transport: diapedesis
blood chlorides, excessive: chloridema,
  hyperchloremia
blood circulation: sanguimotory
blood classification: Arneth's,
  Schilling
  See also blood groups
blood clot: thromb-, thrombo-,
  coagulum, embolus, thrombus
  See also coagulation
blood clot, in brain: cerebral
  thrombosis
blood clot defect: athrombia
blood clot formation:
  thromboendocarditis,
  thrombogenesis, thrombokinesis,
  thrombopoiesis, thrombosis
blood clotlike: thromboid
blood clot removal: fibrinolysis,
  thrombectomy
blood clotting: anticoagulant,
  coagulation, coumarin, Factors I-V,
  VII-XIII, fibrin, fibrinogen,
  heparin, prothrombin,
  thromboplastin
blood coagulant: hematopexin
blood coagulation defect:
  thrombopathy
blood components: cryoprecipitate,
  fibrinogen, granulocytes, packed
  red cells, plasma, plasma
  concentrate, plasma fraction,
  immunoglobulins, leukocytes,
  protein fraction
blood condition: -emia
blood containing: sanguiferous,
  sanguineous
blood count: differential, hemogram,
  Schilling's classification

blood cyst: hematocele
blood deficiency: ischemia
blood diseases: afibrinogenemia,
    agranulocytosis, anemia, dysemia,
    erthroblastosis fetalis,
    hematochromatosis, hemophilia,
    hydremia, leukemia,
    lymphocythemia, nosohemia,
    pyemia, sulhemoglobinemia,
    thalassemia, typhohemia
blood drinking: hematophagia
blood dust: hemoconia
blood flow: circulation, hemorrhage,
    hypostasis, menses, menstruation
blood flow, blocked: aeremia,
    aeroemboliam, embolism,
    hemostasis, thrombostasis
blood flow, stopping: angiopressure,
    angiostrophy, astringent,
    hemostat, staunch, styptic,
    tamponade, tourniquet
blood flow, study of: hemodynamics,
    hemorheology
blood flow measurement:
    densitometry
blood flow promoter: emmenagogue,
    hemagogue
blood fluke: Schistosoma
blood formation: hemapoiesis,
    hemogenesis, hemoplastic
blood formation, defective:
    anhematopoiesis, anhematosis,
    dyshematopoiesis
blood granulocytes, decrease:
    agranulocytosis, granulocytopenia
blood groups: ABO, Auberger, Diego,
    Dombrock, Duffy, high-frequency,
    I, Kell, Kidd, Lewis, low-
    frequency, Lutheran, MNS, P, Rh,
    Sutter, Xg, Yt
blood in chest: hemothorax
blood in eye: hyphemia
blood in feces: hemafecia,
    hematochezia
blood infection: bacillemia,
    bacteremia, sepsis

blood injection: transfusion
blood in joint: hemarthrosis
blood in kidneys: hematonephrosis
blood in middle ear:
    hematotympanium
blood in pleural cavity: hemothorax
blood in scrotum: hematoscheocele
blood in semen: hematospermia
blood in sweat: hemathidrosis,
    hematohidrosis
blood in urine: hematocyturia,
    hematuria
bloodless: ischemic
bloodletting: bdellepithecium,
    hematophagus, hemospasia, leech,
    phlebotomy
bloodlike: hematoid, hemoid
blood loss: bleeding, exsanguination,
    hemorrhage, menstruation
blood nourishment deficiency:
    anemotrophy
blood oxygenation: ventilation
blood oxygenation, deficient:
    anoxemia, hypoxemia
blood parasite: sanguicolous
blood pigment: heme, hemoglobin
blood poisoning: bacteremia,
    eclampsia, ichoremia, pyemia,
    sepsis, septicemia, toxemia
blood pressure: arteriotony
blood pressure, high: hypertension
blood pressure, low: hypotension
blood pressure abnormality:
    anisopiesis
blood pressure inducer: pressor
blood pressure lowering: vasodepressor
blood pressure measurement:
    sphygmomanometry
blood producing: hematopoiesis,
    sanguifacient, sanguification,
    sanguinopoietic
blood relationship: consanguinity
blood retention: hematostatic
blood specialist: hematologist
blood spitting: emptysis, hemoptysis
bloodsucker: hematophagus, Hirudo,
    leech, sanguisuga

blood sugar: glucose
blood sugar, abnormal: diabetes,
hyperglycemia, hypoglycemia
blood sugar, absence: aglycemia
blood therapy: hematherapy,
hematophagia, transfusion
blood thickening: pyknemia,
pyknohemia
blood tumor: hematoma,
hemocytoblastoma
blood urea, excess: azotemia, uremia
blood vessel: angi-, angio-, vaso-,
arteriole, artery, capillary, glomus,
vein, venule
See also aorta, artery, lymph
vessels, veins
blood vessel, affecting: vasoactive
blood vessel, enlarged: aneurysm,
hemangiectasis, phlebarteriectasia
blood vessel abnormal: angiopathy,
varicose veins
blood vessel absent: avascular
blood vessel calcification: angiosteosis
blood vessel calculus: angiolith,
arteriolith, phlebolith
blood vessel caliber change:
vasoconstriction, vasodilation,
vasomotion, vasomotory
blood vessel compression: acupressure,
circumclusion
blood vessel constriction:
angiostenosis, angiotension,
vasoconstriction, vasohypertonic
blood vessel constriction, causing:
angiotensin
blood vessel destruction: angiolysis
blood vessel dilation: aneurysm,
angiectasia, angiohypotonia,
angiomegaly, angiotelectasis,
exangia, hemangiectasis,
vasodilation, vasohypotonic
blood vessel disease: aneurysm,
angiohyalenosis, angioneurosis,
angiopathy, angiosis,
angiosynizesis, atherosclerosis,
embolization, fibromuscular
dysplasia, telangiectasia, varicose
veins

blood vessel disease, anorectal:
hemorrhoids
blood vessel displacement: angiectopia
blood vessel examination:
angiocardiography, angiography,
vasography
blood vessel excision: angiectomy,
angioneurectomy
blood vessel formation: angiopoiesis
blood vessel hardening: angiosclerosis,
arteriosclerosis, atherosclerosis
blood vessel inflammation: angiitis,
angiodermatitis, angiotitis,
endangiitis, endarteritis,
endoangiitis, endoarteritis,
endophlebitis, endovasculitis,
microangiitis, periangiitis,
thromboangiitis, vasculitis
blood vessel junction: abouchement
blood vessel ligation: ultraligation
blood vessel-like: angiod
blood vessel obstruction:
angiemphraxis, embolism,
thromboembolism
blood vessel rupture: angiorrhaphy
blood vessels, study of: angiology
blood vessel softening: angiomalacia
blood vessel spasm: angiohypertoma,
angioneurosis, angiospasm,
vasospasm
blood vessel surgery: angioplasty,
angiostomy, angiotomy, bypass,
percutaneous transluminal
coronary angioplasty
blood vessel tumor: angiolipoma,
angioma, angiomyoma,
angiomyosarcoma, angiosarcoma,
endothelioma, hemangioma,
hemangiosarcoma,
hematolymphangioma,
perithelioma, perivasculitis,
telangioma
blood vessel ulceration: angionoma
blood volume increased: hypervolemia
blood volume reduced: hypovolemia,
oligemia, oligohemia

blood waste removed: dialysis
bloody: plethoric, sanguineous
bloody show: menstruation, vaginal
    bleeding
blowing: insufflation
blue: cyan-, cyano-, cerulean, cyanotic
blue baby: cyanosis, tetralogy of
    Fallot, transposition of the great
    vessels
blue blindness: acyanoblepsia,
    acyanopsia, cyanopsia, tritanopia
blue bloater: chronic obstructive
    pulmonary disease
blue in the face: cyanosis
blues: depression
blue spot: macula cerulea
blunt: -tuse, obtund, obtuse
blurred vision: chorioretinitis
blush: erubescence, erythema, rubedo,
    rubescent vasodilation
blushing, fear of: ereuthrophobia,
    erythrophobia
boat-shaped: scapho-, navicular,
    scaphoid
boat-shaped head: cymbocephalic
body: corpo-, somato-, soma
body, affecting all: systemic
body, dead: cadaver, corpse
body, large: hypermorph,
    macrosomatia
body, overdeveloped: gigantism,
    hypermegasoma
body, small: dwarf, hypomorph,
    microsomia, midget, nanocormia
body and mind: psychophysiologic,
    psychosomatic
body build: ectomorph, mesomorph,
    endomorph, Sheldon; pyknic,
    asthenic, athletic, Kretschmer;
    habitus, hypermorph, hypomorph,
    macrosoma, microsoma, physique,
    somatotype
body cavity: abdominal, coelom,
    cranial, oral, peritoneal, pleural,
    thoracic, visceral
body cavity, missing: acelius,
    acelomate

body clock: circadian rhythm
body defect, denial of: anosgnosia
body deformity: camptocormia,
    camptospasm, prosternation
body fluid, excess: edema, plethora
body fluid, increased pH: alkalosis
body fluid, spreading: suffusion
body fluid discharge: bleeding,
    colliquation, defecation, ejaculation,
    hemorrhage, menstruation,
    sweating, tearing, urination
body fluids: bile, blood, cecal fluid,
    cerebrospinal fluid, extracellular,
    gastric juice, ileal fluid, interstitial,
    intracellular, lacrimal, lymph,
    menses, mucus, pancreatic juice,
    perspiration, saliva, semen,
    seminal, serum, succus, sweat,
    synovial, transcellular, urine, water
body framework: skeleton
body function, study of: physiology
body hair: pelage
body hair, loss: alopecia areata, pelade
body heat loss: thermolysis
body height: stature
body language: kinesics
body louse: pediculosis corporis,
    Phthirus pubis
body measurement, science of:
    anthropometry
body movements: abduction,
    adduction, extension, flexion,
    rotation
body movements, study of: kineto-,
    kinematics, kinesiology
body odor: bromhidrosis, hircismus
    See also odor, smell
body pain: somatalgia
body part, artificial: prosthesis
body positions: See positions
body sensations: somatesthesia,
    somesthesia
body steady state: homeostasis
body structure, study of: anatomy
body temperature measurement:
    thermography

body temperature regulation:
thermotaxis
body temperature variation:
pantothermia
body wastes: cacation, defecation,
diarrhea, elimination, excretion,
exhalation, feces, menses, mucus,
perspiration, pus, respiration,
sweat, urination
body weakness: somasthenia,
somatasthenia
boil: anthracia, carbuncle, furuncle
boiling: effervescence
bonding: attachment, chelation,
maternal-infant
bone: osseo-, osteo-, cancellous,
cartilage, collagen, diaphysis,
diploe, epiphysis, marrow, os,
ossicle, osteon
bone, breaking: osteoclasis
bone, dead: sequestrum
bone, long: diaphysis, epiphysis,
metaphysis
bone, refracturing: anarrhexis
bone, small: ossicle, ossiculum
bone, thickened: pachyostosis
bone, tumorlike: osteomatoid
bone, within: intraosseous
bone atrophy: osteotabes
bone bending: osteocampsia
bone bleeding: osteorrhagia
bone cavity: absconsio
bone cell: osteocyte
bone cell, immature: osteoblast
bone cell, large: osteoclast, osteophage
bone death: osteonecrosis,
osteoradionecrosis
bone decay: caries
bone diseases: Albers-Schoenberg
disease, anostosis, eccentro-
osteochondrodysplasia, dysostosis,
Gradenigo syndrome,
melorheostosis, osteitis deformans,
ostemia, osteoarthropathy,
osteopathology, osteopathy,
osteopenia, osteopetrosis,
osteoporosis, osthexia, Paget's
disease, rheostosis

bone displacement: osteectopia,
parallagma
bone dissolution: osteolysis
bone eating: osteophagia
bone end: epiphysis
bone excision: antrectomy,
diaphysectomy, ostearthrotomy,
ostectomy, osteoarthrotomy,
osteoectomy, sequestrectomy,
sequestrotomy
bone formation: ossification,
osteogenesis
bone formation, defective: dysostosis,
osteodystrophy
bone fracture: See fracture
bone fragment: sequestrum
bone fusion: synostosis
bone graft: hetero-osteoplasty
bone growth, abnormal: exostosis,
hyperostosis, hyperparosis,
hypoparosis, lipping, osteophyma,
osteophyte
bone growth area: metaphysis
bone hardening: eburnation,
osteosclerosis
bone incision: osteotomy, periostotomy
bone inflammation: apophysitis,
diaphysitis, endosteitis, endostitis,
epiphysitis, osteitis, ostempyesis,
osteochondritis, osteomyelitis,
osteoperiostitis, osteosynovitis,
panosteitis, parosteitis, periosteitis,
periosteomedullitis,
periosteomyelitis, periostitis,
periostomedullitis, rarefying
osteitis
bone junction: articulation, syntaxis
bonelike: ossiform, osteoid
bone lining: endosteum
bone loss: deossification, osteopenia,
osteoporosis
bone marrow cell: giant cell,
megakaryocyte, megalokaryocyte,
myeloblast, myelocyte, myeloplast,
myeloplax
bone marrow inflammation: myelitis

bone marrow-like: myeloid
bone marrow production: myelogenic, myelopoiesis
bone marrow tumor: plasmacytoma
bone marrow wastings: myeloma, panmyelophthisis, Waldenstrom's macroglobulinemia
bone mineral loss: deossification
bone nutrition: osteotrophy
bone pain: ostealgia, osteocope, osteodynia, osteoneuralgia
bone production: ossification, osteogenesis
bone protuberance: condyle, exostosis
bone realignment: reduction
bone regeneration: osteoanagenesis
bones, abnormal: fabella
bones, brittle: fragilitas ossium, osteopsathyrosis
bones, long: femur, fibula, humerus, radius, tibia, ulna
bones, long, abnormal: ectromelia
bones, study of: osteology
bone sensitivity: simesthesia
bone separation: disarticulation
bone shaft: diaphysis
bone softening: malacosteon, ossifluence, osteohalisteresis, osteolysis, osteomalacia
bone surgery: osteoclasia, osteoplasty, osteostixis, osteosynthesis
bone suture: articulation, junctura, osteorrhaphy, osteosuture
bone tumors: enchondroma, endosteoma, endostoma, endostosis, Ewing's sarcoma, exostosis, fibro-osteoma, myelosarcoma, osteoblastoma, osteocarcinoma, osteocephaloma, osteochondroma, osteocystoma, osteofibroma, osteoma, osteoncus, osteosarcoma, osteospongioma, osteosteatoma, osteotelangiectasia, periostosis
bone union by ligaments: syndesmosis
bone union by muscle: syssarcosis
bony: osseous

border: acies, edge, limbus, margin, margo, membrane, ora, rim
border, surgery of: marginoplasty
boredom: alysosis
boring: perforation, puncture, terebration, trephining
born: nascent
both: ampho-
both sides: amb-, ambi-, amphi-, ambilateral
bottle-shaped: utriform
boundary: limen, membrane
bound together: arthrodesis, synapsis, syndesis
bowel: colon, intestines
bowel disease: *See* colon, duodenum, ileum, intestine
bowel gas: flatus
bowel gas release: crepitus
bowel movement: defecation, diarrhea, elimination, evacuation, excretion, laxation
bowel movement, infrequent: constipation, costiveness, dyschezia, impaction, intestinal obstruction, obstipation, oppilation, proctostasis, stegnosis
bowel movement, painful: dyschezia
bowel movement inducer: aperient, cathartic, fiber, laxative, purgative, roughage
bowlegs: genu varum, gonyectyposis
bowlike structure: arch, arcus
bow-shaped: arcate, arciform, arcuate
boy: male
braces: *See* orthoses
brain: enceph-, encephalo-, allocortex, archipallium, cerebellum, cerebration, cerebrum, corpus collosum, deutencephalon, diencephalon, encephalon, hippocampus, isocortex, medulla oblongata, metencephalon, midbrain, neocortex, neopallium, pallium, paleopallium, pons, rhinencephalon, telencephalon, thalamencephalon, thalamus,

ventricles
See also cerebellum, cranium, head,
skull
brain, absence: amyelencephalia,
anencephaly
brain, embryonic: afterbrain,
diencephalon, epencephalon,
forebrain, hindbrain,
mesencephalon, metencephalon,
midbrain, myelencephalon,
prosencephalon, rhombencephalon,
telencephalon
brain, large: macroencephalia
brain, small: agyria, cretinism,
microencephalon
brain abscess: encephalopyosis,
pyencephalus
brain areas: Broca's, Brodmann's,
motor, Wernicke's
brain atrophy: encephalatrophy
brain bleeding: encephalorrhagia
brain calculus: encephalolith
brain cavity: ventricle
brain convolutions: gyrus, polygyria
brain defect: anencephaly,
atelencephalia, notencephalocele
brain disease, fear of:
meningitophobia
brain diseases: cephalopathy,
cerebropathy, concussion,
encephalocystocele,
encephalomyelopathy,
encephalopathy, encephalosis,
epilepsy, Gerstmann's syndrome,
hydrencephalocele, hydrocephalus,
hydroencephalocele,
hydroencephalus, organic,
porencephalia, psychosis,
schizencephaly
brain examination: cerebroscopy,
electroencephalography,
encephalography
brain fever: meningitis
brain fissure: anfractuosity
brain function, loss of: anergasia
brain hardening: cerebrosclerosis,
encephalosclerosis, sclerencephalia

brain inflammation: arachnoiditis,
cerebritis, cerebromeningitis,
encephalitis, encephalomeningitis,
encephalomyelitis, endocranitis,
hydromeningitis, leptomeningitis,
meningitis, meningoencephalitis,
meningoencephalomyelitis,
meningomyelitis,
pachyleptomeningitis,
pachymeningitis, parencephalitis,
periencephalitis,
periencephalomeningitis,
perimyelitis, peripachymeningitis,
pia-arachnitis, porencephalitis
brainlike: cerebroid, encephaloid
brain membranes: dura mater,
arachnoid, pia mater; ependyma,
leptomeninges, meninges
brain protrusion. cephalocele,
craniocele, encephalocele,
encephalomeningocele,
hydrencephalomeningocele
brain puncture: encephalopuncture
brain removal: decerebration, pithing
brain sand: acervulus, corpora
arenacea, psammoma bodies
brain softening: cerebromalacia,
encephalomalacia, tephromalacia
brain surgery: cerebrotomy,
cingulotomy, lobotomy, topectomy,
trephination
brain surgery technique: stereotaxy
brain tissue, affinity for: cephalotropic
brain tumors: astrocytoma,
cephalhematocele,
craniopharyngioma, encephaloma,
ependynoma, glioblastoma,
hemangioblastoma,
medulloblastoma, meningioma,
oligodendroglioma,
psammocarcinoma, psammoma,
psammosarcoma
brain ventricle, fifth: cavum septi
pellucidi, Duncan's ventricle
brain ventricle, third: diacele,
thalamocoele

brain wave: alpha, beta, delta, theta
brain wave recording:
    electroencephalogram
branched: arborization, ramified,
    ramose, ramulus, ramus
brandy nose: acne rosacea
brassy eye: chalkitis
break: -clasis, -clast, cleft, comminute,
    dieresis, fracture, rupture
breakbone fever: dengue
break down: catabolism, degradation,
    emulsify
break wind: flatus
breast: mamm-, mammo-, mast-,
    masto-, mazo-, mamma, mammary
    gland, pectus
breast, absence: amastia, amazia
breast, large: gynecomastia,
    hypermastia, macromastia,
    mammose, mastoplasia,
    mastoptosis, pendulous
breast, male, milk secretion:
    androgalactozemia
breast, small: hypomastia,
    micromastia, micromazia
breastbone: sternum
breastbone-like: sternoid
breast cyst: galactocele, lactocele
breast development: mammoplasia,
    mastoplasia
breast development at puberty:
    sororiation, thelarche
breast development in men:
    gynecomastia
breast distention: spargosis
breast examination: mammography,
    thermography
breast feed: suckle
breast fluid: colostrum, milk
breast hardening: mastoscirrhus
breast hyperplasia: mazoplasia
breast hypoplasia: mastatrophy
breast incision: mastotomy
breast inflammation: areolitis,
    mammitis, mastadenitis, mastitis,
    paramastitis

breast milk, lack of: agalorrhea
breast milk secretion, lack of:
    agalactia
breast pain: mammalgia, mastalgia,
    mastodynia, mazodynia
breast removal: mammectomy,
    mastectomy
breasts, multiple: multimammae,
    pleomastia, polymastia, polymazia
breast-shaped: mastoid
breast surgery: mammoplasty,
    mammotomy, mastopexy,
    mastoplasty, mazopexy
breast tumors: eccyclomastopathy,
    fibroadenoma, fibrocystic disease,
    galactoma, mastadenoma,
    mastochondroma, mastoncus,
    pneumogalactocele
breast ulcer: masthelcosis
breath: pneo-, halitus
breath, bad: bromopnea, halitosis,
    ozostomia
breathe in: inspiration
breathe in foreign object: aspirate
breathe out: expiration
breathing: -pnea, pneo-, pneuma-,
    pneumato-, spir-, spiro-, Cheyne-
    Stokes, exhalation, inhalation,
    respiration, trepopnea, ventilation
breathing, deep: bathypnea
breathing, rapid: hyperpnea,
    hyperventilation, polypnea,
    tachypnea
breathing, shallow: hypopnea,
    hypoventilation
breathing, slow: bradypnea
breathing cessation: apnea
breathing difficulty: anhelation,
    dyspnea, liparodyspnea,
    pimelorthopnea
breathing mechanism:
    pneumodynamics
breathing sound: stertor, stridor,
    wheeze
breeding, science of: eugenics
bridge: -desma, obturator, pons

bridges, fear of: gephyrophobia
bristlelike: setaceous, setose
brittle bones: osteogenesis imperfecta
broad: eury-, platy-
broadlegged: platycnemia
broken off: clas-
bromine poisoning: bromism,
  bromomania
bronchial bleeding: bronchorrhagia,
  bronchostaxis
bronchial calculus: broncholith
bronchial dilation: bronchiectasis,
  bronchiocele, bronchiolectasis,
  bronchocele, bronchodilation
bronchial diseases: bronchiolitis,
  bronchopathy, bronchopneumonia
bronchial examination:
  bronchography, bronchoscopy
bronchial incision: bronchotomy
bronchial infection: bronchomycosis
bronchial inflammation: bronch-,
  alveolibronchitis, bronchadenitis,
  bronchitis, bronchoadenitis,
  broncholithiasis, mesobronchitis,
  peribronchitis
bronchial narrowing: bronchiarctia,
  bronchiostenosis, bronchostenosis
bronchial origin: bronchiogenic
bronchial paralysis: bronchoplegia
bronchial secretion, excessive:
  bronchorrhea
bronchial spasm: bronchiospasm,
  bronchospasm
bronchial surgery: bronchoplasty,
  bronchorrhaphy, bronchostomy
bronchial suturing: bronchorrhaphy
bronchial swelling: bronchoedema
bronchiole inflammation:
  peribronchiolitis
bronchodilators: albuterol,
  aminophylline, bitolterol,
  dyphylline, ephedrine, epinephrine,
  ethylnorepinephrine, fenoterol,
  ipratropium, isoetharine,
  isoproterenol, metaproterenol,
  oxtriphylline, racepinephrine,
  terbutaline, theophylline

brothers and sisters: siblings
brown lung disease: byssinosis
bruise: contusion, ecchymosis,
  hematoma, hemorrhagic area,
  livedo, petechia, suggillation
bubble formation: effervescence
bubbling: effervescent
bud: blasto-
Buerger's disease: thromboangiitis
  obliterans
bug: bacillus, bacterium, germ,
  microbe, virus
bulb-shaped: bulbiform
bulge, of eyes: proptosis
bulging: torose
bulk: fiber, roughage
bump: concussion, contusion, cyst,
  eminence, tumor, wheal
bumps on skin: erythema nodosum
bundle: fascicle, vinculum
bunion: hallux valgus
burglers, fear of: sclerophobia
buried alive: vivisepulture
buried alive, fear of: taphephobia
burn: ambustion, brush, chemical,
  cremate, electric, first degree,
  flash, friction, heat, inhalation,
  pyretic, radiation, second degree,
  sunburn, thermal, third degree,
  ustus
burn flesh: scald
burn healing promoter: antipyrotic
burning: acrid, byssocausis, caustic,
  moxibustion, pyrotic
burning pain: causalgia, thermalgia
burning sensation: asphalgesia
burn treatment: cautery, keritherapy,
  ustion
burp: eructation, ructus
bursa calculus: bursolith
bursa disease: bursopathy
bursa excision: bursectomy
bursa inflammation: bursitis
burst open: dehiscence
butter: butyr-
butterfly rash: lupus erythematosus,
  rosacea, seborrheic dermatitis

buttocks: pygo-, breech, clunes,
gluteal region, nates, pygal
buttocks, excess fat: steatopygia
buttocks muscles: gluteus maximus,
gluteus medius, gluteus minimus
buttonhole-like: boutonniere
bypass: shunt

C

cadmium disease: cadmiosis
caffeine: theine
caffeine intoxication: caffeinism,
theaism
caisson disease: aeremia,
aeroembolism, aeropathy,
decompression sickness, dysbarism,
nitrogen narcosis
calcium channel blockers: diltiazem,
nifedipine, verapamil
calcium crushing: calculifragous,
lithotriptic
calcium deficiency: acalcerosis,
calcipenia, calciprivia, halisteresis,
hypocalcemia, osteomalacia,
osteoporosis
calcium fixation: calcipexy
calcium formation: calculosis, lithiasis
calcium in blood, excessive: calcemia,
hypercalcemia
calcium in urine: calciuria
calcium in urine, excessive:
hypercalciuria
calcium loss: decalcification
calculus: lith-, -lith, litho-, coniasis,
concrement, concretion, gallstone,
microlith, stone, sympexion
calculus, breaking: lithotripsy,
saxifragrant
calculus, small: microlith
calculus development: lithogenesis,
microlithiasis
calculus preventive: antilithic
calf: gastrocnemius, sura
calf bone: fibula

calf cramp: systremma
callus: helo-, clavus, heloma, keratoma,
tyloma
callus formation: exostosis, poroma,
porosis, tylosis
calmed: sedated
camphor craving: camphoromania
camphor poisoning: camphorism
canal: alveus, aqueduct, canaliculus,
channel, fistula, fossa, groove,
lumen, trench, tube
cancer: carcin-, carcino-, onco-, basal
cell, carcinoma, leukemia,
lymphoma, malignant, neoplasm,
oncology, sarcoma, tumor
See also tumors
cancer, fear of: carcinophobia
cancer, study of: oncology
cancer causing: carcinogen
cancer destroying: carcinolysis
cancer excision: carcinectomy,
carcinomectomy
cancerlike: cancriform, cancroid
cancer producing: carcinogenesis
cancer tests: biopsy, endoscopy,
Papanicolaou smear, Schiller
See also tests
cancer therapy: acivicin, aclaurubicin,
acodazole, acronine, ambomycin,
ametantrone, aminoglutethimide,
amsacrine, anthramycin,
antineoplastic, asparaginase,
azacitidine, azetepa, benzodepa,
bisantrene, bleomycin, busulfan,
calusterone, caracemide,
carbetimer, carboplatin,
carmustine, chlorambucil,
chlorotrianisene, cisplatin,
cyclophosphamide, cytarabine,
dacarbazine, dactinomycin,
daunorubicin, dezaguanine,
diaziquone, diethylstilbestrol,
doxorubicin, duazomycin,
enpromate, epipropidine,
epirubicin, estradiol, estramustine,
estrogens, estrone, etoposide,
fenretinide, floxuridine,
fluorouracil, fluoxymesterone,
flurocitabine,

hydroxyprogesterone,
hydroxyurea, iproplatin, leuprolide,
levothyroxine, liothyronine, liotrix,
lomustine, mechlorethamine,
medroxyprogesterone, megestrol,
melphalan, menogaril,
mercaptopurine, methotrexate,
methyltestosterone, metoprine,
meturedepa, mitocarin, mitomycin,
mitotane, nocodazole, nogalamycin,
oxisuran, peliomycin,
pentamustine, peplomycin,
plicamycin, prednimustine,
procarbazine, pyrazofurin,
riboprine, semustine, simtrazene,
sparsomycin, spiromustine,
spiroplatin, streptonigrin,
streptozocin, talisomycin,
tamoxifen, tegafur, teniposide,
terpxirone, testolactone,
testosterone, thiamiprine,
thioguanine, thiotepa,
thyroglobulin, thyrotropin,
tiazofurin, uracil mustard,
vinblastine, vincristine, vindesine,
zinostatin, zorubicin
cancer ulceration: carcinomelcosis
canker sore: aphthous, stomatitis
cannibalism: anthropophagy
cannula removal: decannulation
canthus: cantho-
canthus excision: canthectomy
canthus inflammation: canthitis
canthus plastic surgery: canthoplasty
canthus surgery: cantholysis,
    canthotomy
canthus suturing: canthorrhaphy
cap: covering, tegmentum
capillary dilation: angiotelectasia,
    capillarectasia, telangiectasia
capillary disease: capillaropathy,
    telangiosis
capillary examination: capillaroscopy
capillary inflammation: capillaritis,
    telangiitis
capillary tumor: telangioma

capsule: caps-
capsule formation: encapsulation
capsule inflammation: capsulitis
capsule surgery: capsuloplasty
capsule suturing: capsulorrhaphy
carbohydrate: -ose, starch, sugar
carbon: anthraco-, -capnia, carbo-
carbon dioxide in blood, decreased:
    acapnia, hypocapnia
carbon dioxide in blood, excessive:
    hypercapnia
carbuncle: anthraco-, anthracia, boil,
    furuncle
cardiac: *See also* heart
cardiac arrest: asystole
cardiospasm: achalasia
caress: contrectation
caries of spine: Pott's disease,
    trachelocrytosis
carotene in blood: carotenemia
carotene in skin: carotenosis cutis
carotene-like: carotenoid
carotid artery pain: carotidynia,
    carotodynia
carpus excision: carpectomy
carrier: vector
    See also communicable diseases
carriers, study of: phorology
cartilage: chondr-, chondri-, chondro-,
    chondral, chondroblast,
    chondrocyte, chondrogen, collagen
cartilage, abnormal development:
    chondrodystrophy
cartilage degeneration: chondrolysis
cartilage disease: chondralloplasia,
    chondrodysplasia, chondronecrosis,
    chondropathology, chondropathy,
    chondroporosis, dyschondroplasia,
    enchondromatosis
cartilage excision: chondrectomy
cartilage formation: cartilaginification,
    chondrogenesis, chondroplasia,
    chondrosis
cartilage inflammation: chondritis,
    chondroepiphysitis
cartilage-like: cartilaginiform,
    cartilaginoid, chondroid

cartilage pain: chondralgia,
chondrodynia
cartilage softening: chondromalacia
cartilage surgery: chondroplasty,
chondrotomy
cartilage tumor: adenochondroma,
chondroadenoma, chondroangioma,
chondroblastoma,
chondrocarcinoma,
chondroendothelioma,
chondrofibroma, chondrolipoma,
chondroma, chondrosarcoma,
ecchondroma, enchondroma
caseous: tyroid
cast: abduction boots, bandage, Cabot,
halo, mold, Risser, spica, turnbuckle
See also orthoses
cast, false: pseudocast
cast off: abrade, slough
castration: desexualization,
emasculation, eviration,
testectomy, unsex, vasectomy
catalepsy-like: cataleptiform,
cataleptoid
cataract, hard: sclerocataracta
cataract treatment:
phacoemulsification, phacolysis
cathartic: laxative, purgative
cats, fear of: ailurophobia,
galeophobia, gatophobia
cats, love of: ailurophilia, galeophilia,
gatophilia
caul: amnion, greater omentum
cauliflower ear: hematoma auris,
othematoma
cause: etiology
caused: evoked, induced
cause unknown: idiopathic
causing abortion: abortifacient
caustic: amyctic, burning, pyrotic
cauterization: byssocausis,
caloripuncture, chemocautery,
electrocautery, galvanocautery,
igniextirpation, ignioperation,
ignipuncture, inustion,
moxibustion, ustion

cavalry bone: adductor muscle
concretion, rider's bone
cavity: alve-, cel-, -cele, coel-, typhlo-,
acetabulum, antrum, areola,
atrium, bursa, camera, caries,
cavitas, cavum, cisterna, coelom,
crypt, depression, excavation,
follicle, loculus, receptaculum,
recess, sac, sinus, space, tooth
decay, ventricle, vestibule
cavity examination: antroscopy
cavity formation: cavitation
cavity measurement: endometry
cavity wall: paries
cecum: typhlo-, cul-de-sac, pouch,
typhlon
cecum calculus: typhlolithiasis
cecum displacement: cecoptosis,
tephyloptosis
cecum distension: typhlectasis
cecum enlargement: typhlomegaly
cecum excision: cecectomy,
typhlectomy
cecum fixation: cecocolopexy, cecopexy,
typhlopexy
cecum incision: cecotomy, typhlotomy
cecum inflammation: cecitis,
pericecitis, typhlenteritis, typhlitis,
typhloenteritis
cecum narrowing: typhlostenosis
cecum reduction: cecoplication
cecum spasm: typhlospasm
cecum surgery: cecocolostomy,
cecoileostomy, cecosigmoidostomy,
cecostomy, typhlostomy,
typhloureterostomy
cecum suturing: cecorrhaphy,
typhlorrhaphy
celiac plexus paralysis: abepithymia
cell: cyt-, -cyte, cyto-, alpha, alveolar,
ameboid, argyrophil, B, basal,
Bergmann's, beta, border, brush,
centrocyte, chief, chromaffin,
Clara, clear, compartment,
corpuscle, cyton, delta, diploid,
endocrine, endothelial, epithelial,
erythrocyte, foam, ganglion, germ,
giant, glial, goblet, hairy, haploid,
hepatic, hilus, histiocyte, Hurthle,

interstitial, islet, juvenile, killer, Kupffer, Langerhans', Langhans' giant, leukocyte, Leydig's, lymphocyte, macrophage, marrow, mast, motor, mucus, muscle, nerve, neuroglial, neuron, nucleolus, nucleus, null, oat, parietal, pause, phalangeal, pigment, prickle, protoplasm, Purkinje, pyramidal, Reed-Sternberg, satellite, Schwann, segmented, seminoma, Sertoli, sickle, smooth muscle, spindle, stellate, stem, supporting, suppressor, T, unit *See also* blood cell

cell, affinity for: cytotropic

cell, glandular: adenocyte

cell, multistainable: polychromatophile

cell, non-nucleated: akaryocyte, erythrocyte, prokaryote

cell, reproductive: androgone, gamete, gonocyte, ovum, sperm

cell, study of: cytology

cell aggregation: neoplasm, nodule, tumor

cell changes: anabolism, anaplasia, catabolism, cytometaplasia, retromorphosis, retroplasia

cell clumping: agglutination, aggregation

cell components: centriole, centrosome, cholesterol, chromosome granules, cytoplasm, DNA, endoplasmic reticulum, enzymes, glycogen, Golgi complex, lipids, lysosomes, microtubules, mitochondria, nucleolus, nucleus, oncogenes, organelle, plasmid, polysomes, proteins, protoplasm, ribosome, RNA

cell destruction: cellulicidal, cytocidal, cytoclasis, cytolysis, cytophagy, cytotoxic, lysis, meronecrosis, necrocytosis, necrosis

cell differentiation, loss of: anaplasia, dedifferentiation

cell division: amitosis, anaphase, cytodieresis, cytokinesis, interphase, meiosis, metaphase, mitosis, prophase, telophase

cell examination: cytoscopy, electron microscopy, microscopy

cell formation: cytogenesis, cytohistogenesis

cell growth, abnormal: dysplasia

cell growth inhibitor: anagocytic

cell inflammation: cellulitis, celluneuritis

cell layers, in embryo: ectoderm, mesoderm, endoderm

cell-like: cytoid

cell origin: cytogenesis

cell processes: meiosis, mitosis, osmosis, phagocytosis, pinocytosis, secretion

cell producing: cytogenous, cytogeny

cell protection: cytophylaxis

cell regression: anaplasia

cell repair: cytothesis

cell rupture: erythrocytorrhexis, erythrorrhexis, plasmatorrhexis, plasmorrhexis

cells, lack of: acellular

cells, self-destruction: autocytolysis

cells, unequal: anisocytosis

cells in urine: cyturia

cell splitting: plasmoschisis

cellulitis: gangrene

cellulose: cellulin, cellulosan, hemicellulose, polysaccharide

center: centrum, core, heart, navel, nucleus, omphalos

center, away from: distal

center, nearest: proximal

centerward: centrad

centesis: abdominocentesis, amniocentesis, arthrocentesis, cardiocentesis, celiocentesis, celioparacentesis, cephalocentesis, colocentesis, culdocentesis, enterocentesis, keratocentesis, paracentesis, pericardiocentesis, peritocentesis, pleurocentesis, pneumocentesis, puncture, thoracentesis, thoracocentesis

central: entad
cephalosporins: cefaclor, cefadroxil,
cefamandole, cefazolin,
cefmenoxime, cefonicid,
cefoperazone, ceforanide,
cefotaxime, cefotetan, cefoxitin,
cefsulodin, ceftazidime,
ceftizoxime, ceftriaxone,
cefuroxime, cephalexin,
cephalothin, cephapirin,
cephradine, moxalactam
cerebellum: paleocerebellum
cerebellum inflammation: cerebellitis
cerebral cortex: pallium
cerebral ventricles, air in:
pneumoventricle
cerebrospinal fluid, increase of:
hydromyelia, hydrorachis
cerebrum: cerebr-
cerebrum cleft: schizogyria
cervix: See also uterus
cervix dilation: metreurysis, Voorhees
bag
cervix excision: cervicetomy,
cuneohysterectomy,
hysterotrachelectomy,
trachelectomy
cervix fixation: collopexy, trachelopexy
cervix incision: trachelotomy
cervix inflammation: cervicitis,
endocervicitis, trachelitis
cervix surgery: tracheloplasty
cervix suturing: trachelorrhaphy
cesspool fever: typhoid fever
chafing: -tripsis, erythema intertrigo,
excoriation, paratripsis
chalky: calcareous
chamber: atrium, camera
change: meta-, -tropia, conversion,
halmatogenesis, metergasis,
mutation
change, abnormal: metaplasia
change, backward: degeneration,
involution
change, fear of: kainophobia,
kainotophobia, neophobia

change of life: climacteric, menopause
change of voice: heterophonia
channel: alve-, alveus, aqueduct,
canaliculus, cut, fossa, groove,
lumen, nerve, trench, tube
channel formation: canalization
characteristic: -an, -ian, diagnostic,
symptomatic, trait
characteristic, variable: varigate
characterized by: -ulent
charley horse: fibromyositis, muscle
cramp
charm: amulet, fetish, talisman
check: arrest, monitor, staunch,
terminate
check-up: physical examination
cheek: bucca-, bucci-, bucco-, mel-,
melo-, bucca, gena, mala
cheekbone: mala, zygoma
cheek cleft: meloschisis
cheek disease: melasma, melonais,
meloncus
cheek inflammation: melitis
cheek muscle: buccinator
cheek plastic surgery: melonoplasty,
meloplasty
cheerful: sanguine
cheese: tyro-
cheeselike: caseous, tyroid
chelating agents: deferoxamine,
edetate sodium, penicillamine,
phytate sodium
chemical peel: chemosurgery
chemical stimuli: chemotaxis,
chemotropism
chest: stetho-, thoraco-, pectoral,
pectus, thorax
chest, abnormal: koilonychia
chest deformity: chonechondrosternon,
pectus carinatum, pectus
excavatum, thoracocyllosis,
thoracocyrtosis
chest fissure: thoracoceloschisis,
thoracogastroschisis
chest incision: thoracectomy,
thoracobronchotomy, thoracotomy

chest muscles: diaphragm, intercostals, latissimus, pectoralis, scalene, semispinalis, serratus, sternocleidomastoid, sternohyoid, transverse

chest pain: acute myocardial infarction, angina, cholecystitis, dissecting aortic aneuryism, hiatus hernia, hyperventilation, pectoralgia, pericarditis, pleuralgia, pleurodynia, pneumothorax, precardialgia, pulmonary embolus, thoracalgia, thoracodynia

chest puncture: pleurocentesis, thoracentesis, thoracocentesis

chest regions: anterior, posterior, lateral; clavicular, infraclavicular, supraclavicular, mammary, inframammary, sternal; scapular, infrascapular, interscapular, suprascapular; precordial

chest sound: bronchophony, capriloquism, crepitation, egophony, pectoriloquy, pectorophony, rale, rattle, rhonchus, tracheophony, tragophony

chest sounds, instrument: stethoscope

chest spasm: stethospasm

chest surgery: thoracocautery, thoracostomy

chest wound: traumatopnea

chew: masticate

chew, inability to: amastia

chewing, excessive: fletcherism

chicken breast: pectus carinatum

chickenpox: varicella

chilblain: frostbite, kibe, pernio

child: baby, infant, issue, neonate, newborn, offspring

childbearing: pregnancy, texis

childbed: puerperium

childbed fever: puerperal fever

childbirth: accouchement, confinement, delivery, labor, lying-in, parturition, tocus
See also delivery, labor

childbirth, after: postpartum, puerperium

childbirth, before: antepartum

childbirth, diseases after: eclampsia, puerperal fever, sepsis

childbirth, fear of: maieusiophobia, tocophobia

childbirth, normal: eutocia

childbirth, rapid: oxytocin

childbirth methods: Bradley, Lamaze, natural, psychoprophylactic, Read

childbirth specialist: perinatologist

childless: nullipara

childlike: puerile

children: pedia-, siblings

children, specialist: pediatrician, pediatrist, pedologist

children, study of: pediatrics

children, treatment of: pediatry

chill: ague, algor, rigor

chin: genion, mentum, pogonion

chin, beneath: submental

chin plastic surgery: mentoplasty

chisel-shaped: scalpriform

chloride in blood, reduced: chloropenia, hypochloremia

chloride in urine, reduced: hypochloruria

chloride loss: chloroprivic

chlorides in blood, excessive: chloridema, hyperchloremia

chlorides in urine, excessive: chloriduria, hyperchloruria

chlorine: -chloric

choked disk: papilledema

choking: Heimlich maneuver

choking, fear of: pnigophobia

cholera, fear of: cholerophobia

cholera-like: choleriform, choleroid

cholera producing: cholerigenous

cholesterol, bad: low density lipoprotein

cholesterol, decreased: hypocholesteremia

cholesterol, good: high density lipoprotein

choleresterol deposition, excessive:
cholesterolosis
choleresterol in blood, excessive:
cholesterolemia,
hypercholesterolemia
choleresterol in urine: cholesterinuria,
cholesteroluria
cholesterol production:
cholesterolopoiesis
cholinesterase inhibitors: aceclidine,
ambenonium, bethanechol,
carbachol, demecarium,
dexpanthenol, echothiophate,
edrophonium, isoflurophate,
malathion, methacholine,
neostigmine, physostigmine,
pilocarpine, pyridostigmine
cholineresterase reactivator:
obidoxime, pralidoxime
chorealike: choreiform
chorion development: choriogenesis
chorion inflammation: chorionitis
chorion tumors: chorioadenoma,
chorioangioma, choriocarcinoma,
chorioma, deciduoma, placentoma,
syncytioma
Christmas disease: hemophilia B
Christmas factor: Factor IX
chromosomes: autosome, centromere,
chromatid, chromatin,
euchromatin, euploidy,
heterochromatin
chromosomes, abnormal: acrocentric,
aneuploidy, Christchurch,
heptaploid, hexaploid, hyperploidy,
hypoploidy, monosomy, octaploid,
pentaploid, Philadelphia,
polyploidy, polysomy,
submetacentric, telocentric,
triploid, trisomy
chronic: habitual, inveterate
chyle: chyl-, chyli-, chylo-
chyle, carrying: chyliferous,
chylophoric
chyle, excessive: hyperchylia,
polychylia

chyle, lack of: achylia, hypochylia,
oligochylia
chyle formation: chylifacient,
chylifactive, chylification,
chylopoiesis
chyle in blood: chylemia
chyle in heart: chylopericardium
chyle in mediastinum:
chylomediastinum
chyle in peritoneum: chyloperitoneum
chyle in pleural cavity: chylothorax
chyle in testes: chylocele
chyle in urine: chyluria
chylelike: chyliform, chyloid
chyme: pulp
chyme, lack of: oligochymia
ciliary body: cyclo-
ciliary body incision: cyclicotomy,
cyclicotomy, cyclotomy
ciliary body inflammation: cyclitis,
cycloceratitis, cyclochoroiditis,
cyclokeratitis
ciliary body paralysis: cycloplegia
circlelike: cycloid
circular: annular, bulbous, circinate,
discoid, globular, obicular,
perimetric, recurrent, round,
spherical
circumcision: peritomy
clap: gonorrhea
class: -type
classification: Angle's, biotaxis,
Caldwell-Moloy pelvic, Denver,
Dukes', grading, horizon, Killip,
Lancefield, New York Heart
Association, pelvic, Runyon,
staging, taxonomy, TNM, triage,
typing
clavicle: cleid-, cleido-
clawfoot: pes cavus
clawhand: main en griffe
clean, compulsion to: ablutomania
cleansing: abstergent, catharsis,
depuration, detergent, detersive,
purging, purification
clear: hyaline, lucid, pellucid,
transparent

cleavage: bifurcation, fission, fissure, fracture, rupture, section, segmentation

cleft: schisto-, bifid, cleavage, division, fissure, groove, scissura, sulcus, trench

cleft lip: cheiloschisis, harelip

cleft palate: staphyloschisis, uraniscochasma, uranoschisis

cleft palate surgery: palatoplasty, staphyloplasty, uraniscoplasty, uranoplasty

cleft palate suturing: palatorrhaphy, staphylorrhaphy, uraniscorrhaphy, uranorrhaphy, uranostaphylorrhaphy, velosynthesis

clefts, multiple: trifid

clench, of teeth: bruxism, odontoprisis

climate, life and: bioclimatology

climate therapy: climatotherapy

clitoris: membrum muliebre

clitoris, double: diphallus

clitoris disease: clitorism

clitoris enlargement: cliterimegaly

clitoris excision: clitoridectomy

clitoris incision: clitorotomy

clitoris inflammation: clitoriditis, clitoritis

clitoris surgery: clitoroplasty

clogging: congestion, obstruction

closed: atreto-, blocked, impacted, impatent, imperforate, obstructed, obturated, obturator, occluded

clot: coagulation, coagulum, thrombus

clotted: coagulated, grumose, precipitated

cloudiness, of urine: nebula

clouding: opacification

cloudy: fuliginous, opaque, turbid, turbidity, viscid

cloudy, measurement: turbidimetry

cloven spine: spina bifida

club foot: calcaneocavus, calcaneovalgus, cyllosis, equinovarus, kyllosis, pes contorus, reel foot, talipes

clubhand: talipomanus

club-shaped: clavate

clump: acervuline, agglutinate, aggregate, collection, colony, grouping, mass

clumping, cause of: agglutinin, agglutinogen

clumsy: sinistrous

cluster: accumulation, array, conglomerate, nidus

coagulated: thrombosed

coagulation: blood clotting, electrocoagulation, hematopexis, inopexia, photocoagulation
See also blood clot

coagulation disorders: angiohemophilia, Bernard-Soulier syndrome, disseminated intravascular coagulation, hemophilia, von Willebrand's disease

coagulation factors: Factors I-V, VII-XIII, fibrinogen, prothrombin, thromboplastin

coagulation factors, deficiency: afibrinogenemia, hypoprothrombinemia

coagulation preventive: anticoagulant, antithrombin, antithromboplastin, coumarin, heparin, protein C

coat: corium, covering, dermis, epidermis, lamina, membrane

cobweblike: araneous

cocaine addiction: cocainism, cocainomania

cocaine analgesia: cocainization

coccyx: coccyg-, coccygo-

coccyx excision: coccygectomy

coccyx pain: coccyalgia, coccydynia, coccygodynia

cochlea inflammation: cochleitis, cochlitis

coil: convolution, eiloid, helix, intrauterine device, spiral, whorl

coin-shaped: nummular

cold: cry-, crymo-, cryo-, algid, algor, frigid

cold, common: coryza, influenza,
 rhinitis
cold, fear of: cheimaphobia,
 psychrophobia
cold, pain from: cryalgesia,
 crymodynia, psychroalgia
cold, preference for: crymophilic,
 cryophilic, psychrophilic
cold air bath: cryoaerotherapy
cold-blooded: allotherm, poikilotherm
cold hands and feet: acroasphyxia,
 acrocyanosis, acrohypothermy,
 chilblain, pernio, Raynaud's sign
cold perception: rhigosis
cold perception, loss of: cryanesthesia
cold producing: algogenic
cold resistance: crymophylactic,
 cryophylactic, cryotolerant
cold sensation: psychroesthesia
cold sensitivity: cryesthesia
cold sore: Herpes simplex
cold storage: cryobank,
 cryopreservation
cold treatment: crymotherapy,
 cryosurgery, cryotherapy,
 frigotherapy, psychrotherapy
collagen diseases: alkaptonuria,
 ankylosing spondylitis,
 disseminated lupus erythematosus,
 homocystinuria, polyarteritis
 nodosa, scleroderma
 See also connective tissue
collarbone: clavicle
colliculus seminalis: verumontanum
colliculus seminalis inflammation:
 colliculitis, verumontanitis
colliculus seminalis removal:
 colliculectomy
colloidal suspension: emulsoid,
 suspensoid
colon: colo-, colon-, -colon, -colonic
 See also intestine
colon, blind: appendix vermiformis
colon, dilated: Hirschsprung's disease,
 megacolon
colon, long: dolichocolon,
 dolichosigmoid

colon, sacs in: diverticulosis
colon, small: microcolon
colon bleeding: colonorrhagia
colon diseases: adenomatous polyps,
 colonopathy, diverticulosis
colon distension: colauxe
colon examination: colonoscopy,
 coloscopy
colon excision: colectomy,
 coloproctectomy
colon fixation: colofixation,
 colohepatopexy, colonopexy,
 colopexy
colon incision: colotomy
colon inflammation: colitis,
 coloenteritis, coloproctitis,
 colorectitis, Crohn's disease,
 diverticulitis, endocolitis,
 enterocolitis, exocolitis, irritable
 bowel syndrome, paracolitis,
 pericolitis, serocolitis, spastic colon,
 ulcerative colitis
colon irrigation: coloclysis, enteroclysis
colon opening: colostomy
colon pain: coalgia, colonalgia
colon prolapse: coloptosis
colon puncture: colipuncture,
 colocentesis, colopuncture
colon specialist: proctologist
colon surgery: abdominoperitoneal
 resection, coliplication,
 colocholecystostomy, colocolostomy,
 cololysis, colopexostomy,
 colopexotomy, coloplication,
 coloproctostomy, colorectostomy,
 ectocolostomy
color: chrom-, -chromasia, chromat-,
 chromato-, chromo-, chromatic,
 dye, pigmentation
color, fear of: chromatophobia,
 chromophobia
coloration: -chroia
color blind: -anopia, achloropsia,
 achromatic vision, achromatism,
 achromatopia, achromatopsia,
 acritochromacy, acyanoblepsia,
 acyanopsia, aglaukopsia,
 anerythropsia, anianthinopsy,
 axanthopsia, chloropsia,

chromatelopsia, chromatopsia,
chromopsia, cyanopsia, daltonism,
deuteranopia, dichromasy,
dichromatism, dichromatopsia,
dyschromatopsia, erythropsia,
hemichromatopsia, ianthinopsia,
monoblepsia, monochromatism,
parachromatopsia, protanomalopia,
protanopia, tritanomalopia,
tritanopia, xanthocyanopsia
  See also eye, vision
color change: allochroism,
  allochromasia
color difference: heterochromia
colorless: achromatic, albinism,
  pantachromatic, photism
color sensation: -phose, chromesthesia,
  chromophose, photism,
  psychochromesthesia
color vision, normal: euchromatopsy
color vision examination: chromoscopy
coma: comatose, diabetic,
  exanimation, hepatic,
  hypoglycemic, soporose,
  unconscious
coma, light: semicoma, semisopor
coma scale: Glasgow
combination: amalgam
comb-shaped: pectinate
comets, fear of: cometophobia
commissure incision: commissurotomy
common: cen-
communicable diseases: acquired
  immune deficiency syndrome,
  amebiasis, aphthous fever,
  ascariasis, brucellosis, chancroid,
  chickenpox, cholera, diphtheria,
  dysentery, enterobiasis, erysipelas,
  gonorrhea, hepatitis, influenza,
  leprosy, measles, meningitis,
  mononucleosis, mumps, ophthalmia
  neonatorum, pertussis, pneumonia,
  poliomyelitis, psittacosis,
  ringworm, Rocky Mountain
  spotted fever, scabies, scarlet fever,
  smallpox, syphilis, tetanus,
  trachoma, tuberculosis, tularemia,
  typhoid fever, varicella, variola,
  venereal

comparison of structures: morphology
compartmentalized: bilocular, divided,
  sectioned
complaint: ailment, disorder
complete: hol-, holo-, teleo-
complexion, poor: dyschroia
complication: superinfection,
  supervention, suprainfection
compound, breakdown of: analysis,
  catabolism, qualitative analysis,
  quantitative analysis
compress: bandage, pad, pledget
compression: coarctation
compulsion: obsessive-compulsive
  neurosis, gambling, kleptomania,
  psychasthenia, pyromania
compulsory: obligate
concave: amphicelous, procelous
concealed: latent, occult
concentration, equal: isotonic
concentration disorder: hypocathexis,
  psychataxia
conception: fecundation, fertilization,
  impregnation, pregnancy,
  reproduction, syllepsis
concretion: calculus, gallstone, stone,
  sympexion
concussion: commotio
concussion, perception: seisesthesia
condensation: coalescence, distillation,
  evaporation, precipitation
condition: -asia, -esis, -iasis, -ism,
  -osis, -sis, derangement, disease,
  disorder, dysfunction
condyle excision: condylectomy
condyle incision: condylotomy
cone: conus
cone-shaped: conoid, pineal, piniform,
  turbinated
confine: impact, isolate, quarantine,
  restraint
confinement: labor and birth
confinement, fear of: claustrophobia,
  cleisiophobia, cleithrophobia
congenital: ectro-, hereditary, inborn,
  innate, native
  See also hereditary

congenital disorders:
acrocephalosyndactyly,
agenosomia, agnathocephaly, aortic
stenosis, Apert's syndrome, aplastic
cutis congenita, atrial septal
defect, Carpenter's syndrome, cat-
eye syndrome, celosomia, Chediak-
Higashi syndrome, coarctation of
the aorta, cor biloculare, cor
triatriatum, cor triloculare
biatriatum, craniotabes, Crigler-
Najjar syndrome,
cryptomerorachischisis, cyclopia,
Diamond-Blackfan syndrome,
diastematocrania,
diastematomyelia,
diastematopyelia, Down's
syndrome, dyserythropoietic
anemia, Edward's syndrome,
Eisenmenger's tetralogy,
encephalocele, epipygus, epispadias,
erythroblastosis fetalis,
exencephaly, Fordyce disease,
gastroschisis, glaucoma,
hemiplegia, Hirschsprung's disease,
hydrencephalocele, hydrocephalus,
hypoplastic anemia, ichthyosis
congenita, Klippel-Feil syndrome,
lagophthalmos, Larson syndrome,
megacolon, meningocele,
nonspherocytic hemolytic anemia,
Noack's syndrome, notomelus,
oligodactyly, omphalocele, Patau's
syndrome, patent ductus
arteriosus, patent foramen ovale,
persistent cloaca, polycystic
disease, polycystic kidney disease,
prespondylolisthesis, pulmonary
arteriovenus fistula, pulmonic
stenosis, pygomelus, scoliosis, short
neck syndrome, sirenomelia, spina
bifida, subluxation of the hip,
syndactyly, synencephalocele,
syphilis, tetralogy of Fallot,
tricuspid atresia, trisomy 8,
trisomy 13, trisomy 18, trisomy 21,
trisomy 22, transposition of the
great vessels, truncus arteriosus,
Turner's syndrome, ventricular
septal defect, Wolff-
Parkinson-White syndrome
congestion: engorgement, hyperemia,
plethora, turgid
congestion reducer: decongestant
conical: acuminate
conjunctiva disorders: scheroma,
xerophthalmia
conjunctiva edema: chemosis
conjunctiva inflammation:
conjunctivitis, ophthalmia
neonatorum, syndesmitis,
trachoma
conjunctiva surgery: peritectomy,
peritomy, syndectomy
connection: abouchement, adhesion,
anastomosis, annectent, confluence,
copula, isthmus, nexus, relation
connective tissue: aponeurosis, bone,
cartilage, cementum, collagen,
dermis, elastic fibers, epineurium,
epitendineum, epithelium, fat,
fascia, Glisson's capsule, joint
capsule, ligament, mucus, reticular,
teeth, tendon, trabecula
connectice tissue covering: sheath
connective tissue diseases:
alkaptonuria, ankylosing
spondylitis, chondro-
osteodystrophy, cutis laxa,
dermatomyositis, Ehlers-Danlos
syndrome, elastosis,
homocystinuria, lupus, Marfan's
syndrome, mucopolysaccharidosis,
ochronosis, osteogenesis
imperfecta, periarteritis nodosa,
polyarteritis nodosa, polymyositis,
pseudoxanthoma elasticum,
rheumatic fever, rheumatoid
coronary arteritis, scleroderma
connective tissue edema: anasarca,
hyposarca
connective tissue inflammation:
cellulitis, desmosis, panniculitis,
paratyphlitis, peridentitis,
periodontitis, peritendinitis,
peritenonitis, phlegmon, Tietze's
syndrome

connective tissue inflammation, study
of: rheumatology
connective tissue layer: adventitia
tunic
connective tissue origin: desmogenous
connective tissue surgery:
fibromyomectomy, fibromyotomy
connective tissue tumors:
adenofibroma, adenomyosarcoma,
adipofibroma, chondroma,
desmoma, desmoneoplasm,
fibroblastoma, fibrochondroma,
fibrocyst, fibroma, fibromyoma,
fibro-osteoma, fibrosarcoma,
myxoma, neurofibroma,
pseudoneuroma, sarcoma,
syndesmoma
consciousness: apperception,
awareness, perception
consciousness, altered: akinetic
mutism, chronic vegetative state,
coma, concussion, confusion,
dilirium, hypoglycemia, ischemia,
locked-in syndrome, neurolepsis,
seizure, stupor, syncope
consciousness, below: subconscious,
subliminal
consciousness, loss: catalepsy
constipation: costiveness, dyschezia,
impaction, obstipation, oppilation,
proctostasis, stegnosis
constipation corrective: cathartic,
laxative, roughage
constipation producing: analgesics,
anesthetics, antacids,
anticholinergics, anticonvulsants,
antidepressives, diuretics,
emplastic, ganglionic blockers,
hypotensives, opiates,
psychotherapeutics
constriction: atresia, coarctation,
narrowing, phimosis, stegnosis,
stenochoria, stenosis, strangulation
constriction sensation:
strangalesthesia, zonesthesia
constrictor: sphincter, tourniquet

consumption: tuberculosis
contact: apposition, contiguity,
juxtaposition
contageous diseases: See
communicable diseases
container: ampule, flask, syringe, test
tube, vial
See also medicinals
contamination: adulteration,
contagion, degradation, impurity,
pollution, vitiation
contamination, fear of:
molysmophobia, mysophobia
contraceptives: cervical cap, coitus
interruptus, condom, diaphragm,
intrauterine device, oral
contraceptive, pessary, rhythm
method, spermatocide, sponge,
sterilization, tubal ligation,
vasectomy
contractions: anastalis, astringent,
compression, concentration,
fibrillation, peristalsis, tension
contrary: re-
contusion: See bruise
convalescence: cure, recovery,
recuperation, rehabilitation,
remediation, restoration
convert: metabolize, mutate, sublimate
convex: pulvinate
convolution: anfractuous, coil, gyrus,
helix, spiral, whorl
convolutions, excess: polygyria
convulsion, after: postictal, spasm
convulsion causing: eclamptogenic
convulsions: diabetic, eclampsia,
epilepsy, hysteria, intracranial
hemorrhage, tetanus, uremic
convulsion therapy: acetazolamide,
amobarbital, anticonvulsant,
carbamazepine, clonazepam,
clorazepate, diazepam, divalproex,
ethosuximide, ethotoin, lorazepam,
magnesium sulfate, mephenytoin,
mephobarbital, metharbital,
methsuximide, nitrazepam,
paraldehyde, paramethadione,
pentobarbital, phenobarbital,

phensuximide, phenytoin,
primidone, secobarbital,
trimethadione, valproic acid
cooling agent: algefacient, refrigerant
cooperation: coordination, fusion,
synergy
coordination, abnormal: asynergy,
dyssynergy, hyposynergy
copper deficiency: Menkes kinky hair
syndrome
copper toxicity: chalcosis, Wilson's
disease
cord: chord-, chorda, filament, sinew,
tendon
cord excision: chordectomy
cord inflammation: chorditis, corditis,
funiculitis
corn: callus, clavus, heloma
cornea: cerato-, kerat-, kerato-
See also eye
cornea, small: microcornea
cornea bleeding: keratohemia
cornea diseases: Fuch's dystrophy,
hypopyon ulcer, Hutchinson's
patch, keratoconus, keratomyocosis,
keratopathy, salmon patch
cornea enlargement: keratoconus,
keratoglobus, macrocornia,
megalocornea
cornea examination: keratoscopy
cornea excision: keratectomy
cornea hernia: keratectasia,
keratocele, keratorus, keratotorus,
staphyloma
cornea incision: keratotomy,
kerectomy
cornea inflammation: corneitis,
corneoiritis, keratitis,
keratoconjunctivitis, keratoiritis,
keratoscleritis
cornea opacity: albugo, embryotoxon,
keratoleukoma, leukoma, nebula,
nubecula
cornea puncture: keratocentesis
cornea replacement:
prosthokeratoplasty

cornea rupture: keratorrhexis
cornea softening: keratomalacia
cornea surgery: apotripsis,
keratoleptynsis, keratonyxis,
keratoplasty
cornea ulceration: argema,
keratohelcosis
cornea vascular tissue: pannus
cornea wrinkle: rhitidosis, rhytidosis,
rutidosis, rytidosis
corn removal: helotomy
correct: ortho-, rectify, remedy,
straighten
corrosive: caustic, diabrosis, escharotic
cosmetic sensitivity: exfoliative
cheilitis
cosmetic surgery: plastic surgery,
rhinoplasty, rhytidectomy,
rhytidoplasty
costochondrial cartilage inflammation:
Tietze's syndrome
cot death: sudden infant death
syndrome
cough: pertussis, tussis, whooping
cough
cough preventive: antitussive
cough therapy: antitussive,
chlophedianol, codeine,
dextromethorphan,
diphenhydramine, hydrocodone,
hydromorphone, methadone,
morphine
cough up blood: hemoptysis
count, impulse to: arithmomania
count, inability to: anarithmia
counteract: ant-, anti-
counterirritant: acupuncture,
aquapuncture, cataplasm, caustics,
cupping, escharotics, moxibustion,
mustard plaster, poultice,
revulsant, rubefacient, Scotch
douche, urticat, vesicant
covering: adventitia, cap, dressing,
epiglottis, involucrum, lorica,
membrane, obducent, obturator,
operculum, sheath, tectorium,
tectum, tegmen, tegmentum,
tegument

Cowper's glands inflammation:
   antiprostatitis, cowperitis
cowpox: vaccinia
crabs: body louse, morpion, pediculosis,
   Phthirus pubis
crack: cleft, crevice, fissure, groove,
   interstice, rhagade, rima, slit,
   stria, sulcus
cracklike: rhagadiform
crackling: crepitation, decrepitation,
   rales
cradle: arculus
cradle cap: seborrhic dermatitis
cramps: algospasm, colic,
   dysmenorrhea, spasms, systremma
cranial nerves: olfactory, optic,
   oculomotor, trochlear, trigeminal,
   abducens, facial, vestibulocochlear,
   glossopharyngeal, vagus, accessory,
   hypoglossal
cranium: cranio-, calvaria, occiput,
   sinciput, skull
   See also face, head, skull
cranium, abnormal: acrania
cranium, boat-shaped: scaphocephaly,
   tectocephaly
cranium, narrow: stenocephaly
cranium, pus in: pyocephalus
cranium disease: craniopathy,
   craniorachischisis, craniosynostosis
cranium examination: craniotonoscopy
cranium puncture: cephalocentesis,
   craniopuncture
crater: ulcer
craving: -phagia, -philia
craving, abnormal: parepithymia,
   parorexia
craving, alcohol: alcoholophilic,
   narcomania
crazy bone: olecranon
crease: furrow, groove, plication,
   raphe, ridge, ruga, rugose
creatine in blood, excessive:
   creatinemia
creatine in urine, excessive:
   creatinuria

creeping: serpiginous
creeping eruption: cutaneous larva
   migrans
cremation: tephrosis
crescent-shaped: falciform, lunula,
   semilunar
crescent-shaped cartilage: meniscus
crest: crista, head, projection, ridge
crib death: sudden infant death
   syndrome
cribriform: ethmoid
cricoid cartilage excision:
   cricoidectomy
cricoid cartilage pain: cricoidynia
cricoid cartilage incision:
   cricothyreotomy, cricotomy,
   cricotracheotomy
crisis: acme, apostasis, emergency
criticism, fear of: enissophobia
crocodile tears syndrome: gustatory-
   lacrimal reflex
cross-breeding: hybridization
cross-dressing: transvestism
cross-eyed: esotropia, strabismus
crossing: chiasm, decussation,
   interlacing
cross-section: transection
cross-shaped: cruciate, cruciform
crosswise: transverse
croup: angina trachealis, exudative
   angina, laryngostasis,
   laryngotracheobronchitis
croup, false: laryngismus stridulus,
   pseudocroup
crowds, fear of: demophobia,
   ochlophobia
crownlike: corona, coronoid
cruelty: sadism, tyrannism
crush: -clasia, -tripsy, clasmatosis,
   fragment, pulverize, quassation,
   triturate
crust: coating, incrustation, mantle,
   scab, slough
crying: epiphora, illacrimation,
   ululation
crypt: depression, odontobothrion, pit,
   slit

crypt calculus: cryptalith
crypt excision: cryptectomy
crypt inflammation: cryptitis
crystalline: hyaline
crystals in urine: crystalluria
C section: cesarean section
Cuban itch: alastrim, amaas, variola
   minor
culture media: agar, beef infusion,
   Bennett, blood, Bordet-Gengou,
   brain-heart infusion, brilliant
   green, broth, Cary and Blair
   holding medium, Czapek, dextrose,
   Dubos', Dulaney, eosin-methylene
   blue, Feeley-Gorman, Hickey and
   Tresner, infusion, Jones-Kendrick,
   Kliger iron, Littman oxgall,
   Lombard-Dowell, MacConkey's,
   Martin's nutrient, Mueller-Hinton,
   phenol red, Sabhi, Sabouraud,
   Staib, Thayer-Martin, Todd-
   Hewitt, trypticase soy, Wickerham,
   Wilkins-Chalgren, Wolin-Bevis,
   yeast extract, zein
cupping glass: cucurbitula, cup,
   ventouse
cup-shaped: caliculus, calix,
   calyciform, cotyloid, scyphoid
curative: healing, remedial, salutary,
   sanative, therapeutic
curdled: coagulated
cure: antidote, elixir, heal, recovery,
   recuperation, remediation, remedy,
   restoration
cure, natural: physiatrics
cure-all: panacea, panchreston
curvature: hettocyrtosis
curve outward: excurvature
cushion-shaped: pulvinate
cut: -tome, dissection, incision, injury,
   laceration, lance, section, wound
cutaneous disorders: *See* skin
cuticle: eponychium
cut into: discission, incision
cut out: ablate, abscission, excision,
   extirpation, resect

cut teeth: odontiasis, teething
cutting: -tome, lancinating
cutting edges: saw, sectorial, teeth
cycle: cyclo-
cycles: biorhythm, bipolar disease,
   cardiac, circadian rhythm,
   genesial, Kreb's, menstrual,
   respiratory, sleep
cylinder-shaped: cylindroid
cyst: cyst-, cysti-, cystido-, cysto-
cyst, few: oligocystic
cystlike: cystiform, cystoid,
   cystomorphous
cyst of pus: pyocyst, pyopneumocyst
cyst of urine: urinoma, uroncus
cysts: Epstein's pearls
cysts, watery: hydroma, hygroma

D

daily: diurnal, quotidian
dampness, fear of: hygrophobia
dancing: saltation
dancing mania: chorea, choreomania,
   choromania, tigretier
dandruff: furfur, pityriasis capitis,
   seborrhea
dandy fever: dengue
dangerous: pernicious
darkness: scoto-
darkness, fear of: noctiphobia,
   nyctophobia, scotophobia
darkness, love of: nyctophilia,
   scotophilia
darkness, sensation of: aphose,
   centraphose
dartlike: spicular
dawn, fear of: eosophobia
day blindness: hemeralopia
daydreaming: oneirism, phantasy
daylight, fear of: phengophobia
dead: necro-, thanato-
dead at birth: stillborn
dead body: cadaver, corpse
dead body, desire for: necrophilia

dead body, examination of: autopsy, necropsy, necroscopy, necrotomy, obduction, postmortem, thanatopsy
dead body, fear of: necrophobia, thanatophobia
dead matter, living on: metatrophic, saprophytic, saprozoic
deaf mute: surdomute
deafness: anacroasia, anacusis, anakusis, conductive, Mondini, otosclerosis, sensorineural, surditas
See also hearing
deafness, partial: hemianacusia
death: necro-, thanato-, apobiosis, mors
death, after: posthumous, postmortem, postnecrotic
death, before: antemortem
death, desire for: necromania, necrophilism, suicidal, thanatomania
death, fear of: necrophobia, thanatophobia
death, preoccupation: thanatopsis
death, resembling: thanatoid
death, science of: necrology, thanatology
death-causing: apocarteresis, lethal, suicide
death instinct: thanatos
death of cells: abiotrophy, gangrene, necrosis
death rate: mortality
death sign: thanatognomonic
death struggle: agony
death with dignity: agathanasia, euthanasia
debilitated: asthenia, impaired, inanition, weakness
debility: atony
decay: sapro-, atrophy, decomposition, degenerate, putrescence, putrid
decay causing: pythogenic
decisions, inability to make: aphronia
decomposition: fermentation, lysis, putrefaction

decompression sickness: aeremia, aeroembolism, aeropathy, caisson disease, dysbarism, nitrogen narcosis
decompression tank: hyperbaric chamber
decreased: -penia
deep: batho-, bathy-
deep-seated: profunda
deep sensibility: bathyesthesia
deep sensibility, excessive: bathyhyperesthesia
deep sensibility, loss of: bathyanesthesia, bathyhypesthesia
deerfly fever: tularemia
defecation: cacation, dejecta, excrement, stool
defecation, fear of: defecalgesiophobia, rhypophobia, scatophobia
defecation, uncontrolled: encopresis, incontinence
defect: flaw, imperfection, vitium
defense mechanism: antibody, antigen, compensation, conversion, displacement, dissociation, immunology, rationalization, reaction formation, repression, sublimation
deficiency disease: ariboflavinosis, avitaminosis, Barlow's, beriberi, biotin deficiency syndrome, folic acid deficiency anemia, fucosidosis, infantile scurvy, kwashiorkor, mucopolysaccharidosis, pellagra, rickets, scurvy
See also malabsorption diseases, metabolism diseases, vitamin deficiency
deficient: hypo-, oligo-, -penia
deflect: refract
deformed: pero-, terato-, paraplastic
deformity: anomaly, birth defect, congenital anomaly, malformation, malfunction
deformity, fear of: dysmorphophobia
deformity correction: redressement

degeneration: abiotrophy, atrophy, deterioration, devolution, dystrophy, hypotrophy

degenerative diseases: ataxia telangiectasia, beta-lipoproteinemia, familial ataxia, Friedreich's ataxia, hepatolenticular, olivopontocerebellar, osteoarthritis, osteoarthrosis, parkinsonism, spinocerebellar

dejection: depression

delayed: mentally deficient, retarded

Delhi boil: cutaneous leishmaniasis

delicate: lepto-

delirium: typhomania

delirium, from fever: pyretotyphosis

delirium tremens: potomania, tromomania

delivery, abdominal: cesarean section, laparotrachelotomy

delivery, abnormal: asynclitism, breech, brow, crossbirth, footling, obliquity, transverse

delivery, difficult: dystocia

delivery, surgery for: episiotomy, hebosteotomy, hebotomy, pelvioplasty, pubiotomy, symphysectomy, symphysiectomy, symphysiotomy, synchondrotomy

delivery date: Naegele's rule

delusion: cacodemonomania, callomania, galeanthropy, hallucination, illusion, megalomania, micromania, necromimesis, nihilism, plutomania, zoanthropy

dementia: Alzheimer's disease, Creutzfeldt-Jakob disease, obstructive hydrocephalus, paresis, Pick's disease, senile psychosis, Wilson's disease
See also manias, mental diseases, senility

demons, fear of: demonophobia

demons, possessed by: demonomania, demonopathy

dense: pycno-, pykno-

density decrease: rarefaction

dentin formation: dentification, dentinoblast, dentinogenic

dentin inflammation: dentitis

dentinlike: dentoid

dentist, fear of: odontophobia

dentistry: endodontics, exodontics, maxillofacial surgery, odontiatria, odontology, odontotechny, oral surgery, orthodontics, pedodontics, periodontics, prosthetic, prosthodontics, rhizodontropy

deodorant: anhidrotic, antibromic, antihidrotic, antiperspirant, antisudorific

dependence: addiction, anaclisis

deposit: precipitate, sediment

depression: abaissement, acedia, alveolus, cavity, crevice, dejection, dysphoria, excavation, fossa, fovea, hollow, hospitalism, impression, melancholy, pit, recess, socket, tristimania, trough, vallecula

depression therapy: adinazolam, alaproclate, aletamine, amitriptyline, amoxapine, antidepressant, aptazapine, azepindole, bipenamol, bupropion, butriptyline, caroxazone, cidoxepin, clomipramine, cyclindole, cyprolidol, desipramine, dibenzepin, dioxadrol, doxepin, encyprate, fantridone, fenmetramide, fluoxetine, gamfexine, imafen, imipramine, isocarboxazid, lortalamine, maprotiline, melitracen, modaline, napactadine, nomifensine, nortriptyline, octriptyline, oxaprotiline, oxtpertine, phenelzine, pirandamine, pridefine, protriptyline, rolicyprine, sertraline, sulpiride, tametraline, tandamine, thiazesim, thozalinome, tranylcypromine, trazodone, trimipramine, viloxazine, zimeldine, zometapine

depth: batho-, bathy-
depths, fear of: bathophobia
dermatology: *See* skin
descent: descensus, heredity,
    procidentia, ptosis
desert fever: coccidioidomycosis
destroy: ablate, disinfect, lyse,
    pulverize
destructive: lyso-, aneretic, lysis
detachment: ablation, abruptio, amotio
deterioration: abalienation, atrophy,
    degeneration, retrogression
developed within: endogenous
development: genesis, morphogenesis,
    phylogenesis
development, abnormal: agenesis,
    aplasia, ateliosis, cacogenesis,
    dysgenesis
development, early: precocious
development, stage of: -blast, blasto-,
    blastocyst, morula, zygote
developmental period: incubation
    period, latent period
deviation: ap-, apo-, -tropia,
    aberration, acatastasia, anomaly,
    deformity, heteromorphous,
    perversion
devil, fear of: demonophobia,
    satanophobia
devil's grip: Bornholm disease,
    epidemic pleurodynia
dextrality: right-handedness
dhobie itch: tinea cruris
diabetes, caused by: diabetogenous
diabetes, type I: insulin-dependent
diabetes, type II: adult-onset,
    noninsulin-dependent
diabetes causing: diabetogenic
diabetes therapy: acetohexamide,
    antidiabetic, buformin,
    chlorpropamide, ciglitazone,
    etoformin, gliamilide, glibornuride,
    gliflumide, glipizide, glyburide,
    glyparamide, insulin, linogliride,
    metformin, tolazamide,
    tolbutamide, tolpyrramide

diagnosis, procedures:
    anaphylodiagnosis, auscultation,
    percussion, physiognosis
    See also tests
diagnosis, uncertain: acatalepsia
diagnostic: diacritic
diagnostic aids: acetylcysteine, amyl
    nitrate, bentiromide, chorionic
    gonadotropin, chromate-51,
    clomiphene, cosyntropin,
    cyanocobalamin, demecarium,
    dexamethasone, diatrizoate
    meglumine, diatrizoate sodium,
    dinoprost, disofenin,
    echothiophate, edrophonium,
    ergonovine, erythrosine, etifenin,
    ferrous citrate, fludrocortisone,
    fluorescein, folate sodium, folic
    acid, gallium-67, glucagon,
    gonadorelin, hydroxocobalamin,
    hydroxypropyl methylcellulose,
    indium-111, inulin, iocetamic acid,
    iodine-131, iodipamide, iopanoic
    acid, iothalamate meglumine,
    ipodate, isoflurophate, krypton-
    81m, levothyroxine, liotrex,
    metrizamide, neostigmine,
    oxytocin, pancrelipase,
    pentagastrin, pentetic acid,
    phenolsulfonphthalein,
    phenylephrine, protirelin,
    selenomethionine, simethicone,
    spironolactone, succimer,
    technetium-99m, thallous chloride,
    thyroglobulin, thyroid, thyrotropin,
    tropicamide, tuberculin,
    tyropanoate, xenon-133
diagnostic tests: *See* tests
diaper rash: candidiasis, candidosis
diaphragm: phren-, phreno-
diaphragm, beneath:
    subdiaphragmatic, subphrenic
diaphragm hernia: diaphragmatocele
diaphragm inflammation:
    diaphragmitis, paraphrenitis
diaphragm pain: diaphragmalgia,
    diaphragmodynia, phrenodynia

diaphragm paralysis: phrenoplegia
diaphragm surgery: phrenocolopexy
diarrhea: cacatory, dysentery
diarrhea causes: bacterial exotoxins, bile acids, dysentery, hormones, intestinal distension, laxatives, neurotransmitters
diarrhea therapy: activated charcoal, aluminum hydroxide, codeine, glycopyrrolate, loperamide, opium, paregoric, polycarbophil, psyllium
dietetic therapy: alimentotherapy, dietotherapy, sitotherapy
diets: balanced, Banting, basic, bland, elimination, fasting, fluid, full liquid, Karell, Kempner's, ketogenic, liquid, Mayo clinic, Moro-Heisler, regular, salt-free, Schemm, Sippy, smooth, soft
different: all-, allo-, hetero-, anarchic
differentiate: distinguish, discriminate
difficult: bary-, dys-, mogi-
digestion: absorption, anabolism, assimilation, eupepsia
digestion, impaired: cacochylia, dyspepsia, hyperpepsia, hypopepsia
digestion, self: autodigestion, autopepsia, autophagia
digestion cessation: apepsia
digestive juices: -chylia
digestive product: chyle, chyme, feces, pulp
digestive secretion, lack of: achlorhydria, achylia
digestive tract: alimentary canal; mouth, pharynx, esophagus, stomach, small intestine (duodenum, jejunum, ileum), large intestine (cecum, colon, rectum), anus
digestive tract, primative: archenteron, archigaster, colenteron, gastrocele
digit: dactyl-, -dactyl, -dactylia, dactylo-, -dactyly, dactyl, dactylus, finger, toe
See also extremities, finger, limb, toe

digit cramp: dactylospasm
digit disease: acrodactyly, acrosclerosis, ainhum
digit fusion: acrosyndactyly, ankylodactyly, dactylion, symphalangism, syndactyly, zydodactyly
digit gangrene: acrosphacelus
digit inflammation: dactylitis, phalangitis
digit pain: dactylocampsodynia
digits, abnormal: acropathy, didactylism, hexadactyly, hyperdactyly, hyperphalangism, hypodactyly, isodactyly, megadactyly, monodactylism, perodactyly, polydactyly, sexdigitate, triphalangia
digits, abnormal flexion: camptodactyly
digits, absence: adactyly, aphalangia, ectrodactyly, oligodactyly
digits, large: dactylomegaly, macrodactyly, megalodactyly, pachydactyly
digits, long: arachnodactyly
digits, odd numbered: imparidatale, perissdactylous
digits, short: brachydactylia
digits, skin induration: sclerodactyly
digits, small: microdactyly
digit surgery: phalangectomy
dilation: distension, ectasia, expansion
dilation, blood vessel: aneurysm
dilation, excessive: parectasis
dilator: mydriatic
diluted: attenuated, comminuted
diminished: hypo-
diphtheria-like: diphtheroid
diphtheria test: Schick
dirt, fear of: mysophobia, rhypophobia, rupophobia
dirt eating: geophagia
disability: impairment
discharge: -rhage, -rhagia, -rrhea, cenosis, emission, excretion, ichor, mucus, orrhorrhea, purulence, pus, rheum, sanies, saniopurulent, sanioserous, suppuration

discharge suppression: epistasis
discoloration, of body tissue:
    ochronosis
disease: -iasis, noso-, path-, patho-,
    -pathic, abnormal, affliction,
    ailment, condition, contagion,
    disability, disorder, dyscrasia,
    dysfunction, infection, mal,
    malady, morbid, morbus, nosology,
    pathologic, pathosis, pestilence,
    plague
    See also communicable diseases,
    infectious diseases
disease, caused by another disease:
    secondary
disease, delusions of: nosomania
disease, fear of: monopathophobia,
    nosophobia, pathophobia
disease, female: gynecopathy
disease, imitation of: malingering,
    pathomimesis, pathomimicry
disease, intensified: anabasis
disease, main: primary
disease, male: andropathy
disease, new: neopathy
disease, opposite to: allopathy
disease, spread of: epidemic,
    infections, pandemic, prosodemic
disease, study of: epidemiology,
    etiology, pathology,
    pathomorphism, semeiosis
disease, unable to produce: avirulent
disease, unknown origin: autopathy,
    idiopathic
disease carrier, study of: phorology
disease causes, study of: etiology
disease classification: nosology,
    nosonomy
diseased: coc-, coci-, coco-
disease decline: catabasis
disease development: nosogenesis,
    pathogenesis, pathogeny
disease from poor nutrition: dystrophy
disease identification: diagnosis,
    differential diagnosis
disease improvement: remission

disease indication: pathognomonic,
    sign, symptom
disease indicator: prodrome
disease onset: prodromal
disease origin: nidus, pathogeny
disease prediction: prognosis
disease predisposition: diathesis,
    procatarxis
disease prevention: isolation,
    prophylaxis, quarantine,
    seroprevention, seroprophylaxis,
    serovaccination, vaccination
disease producing: morbific,
    nosopoietic, pathogenesis, peccant
disease rate: morbidity
disease recurrence: palindromia,
    polyleptic, relapse
disease resistance: defense, immunity
diseases, multiple: polypathic
disease signs, disappearance: apeidosis
disease specialist: pathologist
disease transmitter: fomes,
    pathophoresis
disease treatment: See therapy
disease worsening: recrudescence,
    relapse
disfigurement: deformity
dish face: facies scaphoidea
disinfectants: bensalan, benzoxiquine,
    chlorocresol, cloflucarban,
    clorophene, cresol, dibromsalan,
    fluorosalan. formaldehyde,
    fursalan, glutaral, halazone, ictasol,
    metabromsalan, oxyquinoline,
    phenolate, thiosalan, tibrofan,
    tibromsalan, triclocarban, triclosan
disk inflammation: diskitis, meniscitis
disklike: discoid
disk-shaped: nummular
dislocation: luxation, subluxation
dislocation of joint: abarticulation
dislocation reduction: embole, taxis
disorder: See disease
disorder, fear of: ataxiophobia
disordered: dys-
disorientation: anomie

dispersion: diaeresis
displaced: atopic, ectopic
displaced backward: retroposed, retroversion
displaced forward: proptosis
displacement: dislocation, dystopia, ectopia, luxation
dissimilar: aniso-
dissolution: -lysis, lysis
dissolved: lyo-
distended: dilated, engorged, patulous, ventricose
distended abdomen: meteorism, tympanites
distension: dilated, swelling, turgor
distinguish: differentiate, discriminate
distress: angor, angor animi
diuretics: ambuside, amiloride, azolimine, azosemide, bendroflumethiazide, benzthiazide, brocrinat, bumetanide, chlorothiazide, chlorthalidone, clazolimine, cyclothiazide, ethacrynic acid, etozolin, fenquizone, furosemide, glycerin, hydrochlorothiazide, hydroflumethiazide, indapamide, isosorbide, mannitol, mefruside, methylclothiazide, metolazone, ozolinone, piretanide, polythiazide, quinethazone, spironolactone, triamterene, trichlormethiazide, triflocin, urea
See also antihypertensives
diver's disease: aeremia, aeroembolism, aeropathy, caisson disease, decompression sickness, dysbarism, nitrogen narcosis
divert: bypass, shunt
diverticulum: pouch, sac
diverticulum excision: diverticulectomy
diverticulum inflammation: diverticulitis, peridiverticulitis
divide: bisect, cleavage, dissect, meiosis, mitosis, nullify

division: schizo-, bifurcation, cleft, fission, segmentation
dizziness: disequilibrium, fainting, Gerlier's disease, Meniere's disease, scotodinia, vertigo
dizziness therapy: belladonna, dimenhydrinate, diphenhydramine, hyoscyamine, meclizine, promethazine, scopolamine
doctoring: treatment
dogs, fear of: cynophobia
dolls, fear of: pediophobia
dormant: comatose, latent, topor, torpent
dosage, science of: posology
dotage: senility
dotted: punctate
double: amphi-, bi-, di-, diplo-, bigeminal
double chin: buccula
double-edged: ancipital
double vision: diplopia
doubling: amphi-
down: de-, depressed, prostrate
Down's syndrome: mongolism, trisomy 21
downward: cata-, deorsumduction
downy: pilose
draw back: dorsiduct
drawing: traction
draw off: aspirate, drain
draw toward: odduct, retract
dreams: oneiro-, delusions, illusions, nightmares, paroniria
dreams, analysis of: oneiroscopy, psychoanalysis
dreams, study of: oneirology
dressing: bandage, compress, fomentation, gauze, tourniquet
drill: abaptiston
drink: -posia, addiction, alcoholism, fluid intake, intoxication, potion
drinkable: potable
drinking, fear of: dipsophobia
drive, basic: hunger, respiration, sex, thirst

drive away: -fuge
drooling: sialorrhea, sialozemia
droop: ptosis
drop: -ptosis, descensus, gutta, minim,
    ptosis, procidentia, prolapse
dropsy: anasarca, ascites, edema,
    hydrops
drowsy: somnolent, somnolentia
drug: pharmaco-, antibiotic,
    barbiturate, depressant,
    hallucinogen, hypnotic, medication,
    medicine, narcotic, pharmaceutical,
    psychedelic, sedative, soporific,
    stimulant, tranquilizer
drug, fear of: pharmacophobia
drug, fake: placebo
drug, science of: pharmacognosy
drug, study of: pharmacodynamics,
    pharmacokinetics, pharmacology
drug addiction: pharmacopsychosis
drug against bacteria: antibacterial,
    antibiotic, antimicrobial,
    bactericide, bacteriostat
drug-caused: dermatitis
    medicamentosa
drug container: cachet, capsule, pill,
    wafer
    See also medicinals
drug craving: narcomania,
    pharmacomania
drug habit: dependence
drugist: apothecary, pharmacist,
    pharmacologist
drug mixture for pain: analgesic
    cocktail, lytic cocktail
drug overdose: polypharmacy
drugs, euphoric: cannabis,
    hallucinogen, hashish, heroin, LSD,
    marijuana, mescaline, morphine,
    peyote
drug state: kaif
drugstore: pharmacy
drug treatment: chemotherapy,
    methadone, pharmacotherapy,
    polypharmacy, therapeutics
drunk: alcoholic, inebriated,
    intoxicated

dry: dehydration, desiccate, exsiccate,
    kraurosis, parched, siccant, siccus,
    xerantic, xerosis, xerotes
dry lips: xerocheilia
dry mouth: xerostomia
dry skin: xerosis
duct: canal, tube, vas
duct, dilated: ampulla, cul-de-sac
duct gland: exocrine gland
ductless gland: endocrine gland
dull: bary-, brady-, obtund, obtuse,
    phlegmatic
dullness: ambly-, reduced resonance
dumb: mental retardation, mute
duodenum examination:
    duodenography, duodenoscopy
duodenum excision: duodenectomy,
    duodenopylorectomy
duodenum incision:
    duodenocholedochotomy,
    duodenotomy
duodenum inflammation: duodenitis,
    duodenocholangitis, periduodenitis
    See also intestine
duodenum surgery:
    duodenocholecystostomy,
    duodenoenterostomy,
    duodenoileostomy,
    duodenojejunostomy,
    duodenoplasty, duodenostomy
duodenum suturing: duodenorrhaphy
duplication: dis-
dura mater: pachymenix
dura mater disease:
    pachymeningopathy
dura mater inflammation: duritis,
    duroarachnitis, pachymeningitis,
    perimeningitis
dura mater repair: duraplasty
dust, fear of: amathophobia
dust-causing diseases: anthracosis,
    asbestosis, cituminosis, coniosis,
    lithicosis, pneumoconiosis, silicosis
dust corpuscle: hemoconia
dusting powder: exciccant
dwarf: homunculus, hyponanosoma,
    nanism, nanosomia, nanus

dwarfism: achondroplasia,
    chondrodystrophy, Cockayne's
    syndrome, cretinism, Dubowitz
    syndrome, dyschondrosteosis,
    Morquio's syndrome,
    osteochondrodystrophy, pygmy,
    thanatophoric
dwarflike: nanoid
dye, affinity for acid: acidophil
dyes: acriflavine, alizarin, aniline,
    azalein, azocarmine, cochineal,
    diphenylmethane, eosin, Evans
    blue, fluorescein, fuchsin,
    hematoxylin, ketonimine,
    methylene blue, peonin, rosanilin,
    scarlet red, sulfobromophthalein,
    triphenylmethane, triple, vat, vital
dying: moribund
dysentery: amebiasis, diarrhea
dysentery preventive: antidysentery
dyspnea: pneumatodyspnea
dysuria preventive: antidysuria

E

ear: aur-, ot-, oto-, ala auris, auris,
    pinna, auricle, meatus, tympanic
    membrane, malleus, incus, stapes,
    labyrinth, semicircular canal,
    cochlea
ear, behind: opisthotic, retroauricular
ear, bleeding from: othemorrhagia,
    otorrhagia
ear, inner: labyrinth
ear, large: macrotia
ear, nose, throat doctor:
    otolaryngologist
ear, one: monotic
ear, origin in: otogenous
ear, outer: auricle, concha, pinna
ear, pus in: pyolabyrinthitis,
    pyotorrhea
ear, ringing in: tinnitus
ear, round: periotic
ear, small: microtia

ear, study of: otology, otoneurology
ear abnormality: ankylotia, anotia,
    polyotia, synotia
earache: otalgia, otodynia,
    otoneuralgia
ear depression: scapha, scaphoid fossa
ear discharge: otoblennorrhea,
    otocatarrh, otopyorrhea,
    otorrhagia, otorrhea
ear diseases: cholesteatoma,
    chondrodermatitis nodularis,
    labyrinthine vertigo, Meniere's
    disease, mycomyringitis,
    myringomycosis, othelcosis, otitis
    mycotica, otomyces, otomycosis,
    otopathy, otopyosis, otosclerosis,
    tympanitis
eardrum: myringo-, tympano-,
    myringa, tympanic membrane
eardrum disease: myringomycosis
eardrum excision: myringectomy,
    myringodectomy
eardrum fixation:
    myringostapediopexy
eardrum incision: myringotomy
eardrum inflammation: myringitis,
    myringodermatitis
eardrum rupture: myringorupture
eardrum surgery: myringoplasty
ear dust: otoconia, otolith, statoconia
ear examination: otoscopy
ear fluid: endolymph
ear inflammation: aerotitis, barotitis,
    bullous myringitis, cochleitis,
    cochlitis, labyrinthitis, otitis media,
    otoantritis, panotitis
earlobe edema: othygroma
ear margin: helix
ear noises: sonitus, syrigmus, tinnitus
ear obstruction: otocleisis
ear pain: odynacusis
ear paralysis: otomyasthenia
earpick: auriscope
ear pouch: utricle
ear puncture: auripuncture
ear-shaped: auriform

ear specialist: aurist, otolaryngologist, otologist

ear surgery: labyrinthectomy, labyrinthotomy, otectomy, otonecrectomy, otoplasty, ototomy, stapedectomy, stapediotenotomy, vestibulotomy

ear tumor: otoncus, otopolypus

earwax: cerumen

earwax, excessive: ceruminosis

eat: phag-, phago-, -phagia, -phagy, ingest

eating, fear of: phagophobia

eating disorders: acoria, allotriophagy, anorexia, apastia, bulimia, coprophagy, dumping syndrome, fastidium, geophagia, monophagia, parorexia, pica, polyphagia, obesity, rhypophagy, scatophagy
    See also food, hunger

eating fast: tachyphagia

eating slow: bradyphagia

ecchymosis: See bruise

echolike: resonance

edema: anasarca, dropsy, hydrops

edema therapy: antihydropic, diuretic
    See also diuretics

edge: border, limbus, lip, margin, rim

edges, two: ancipital

effect: -ergy

egg: oo-, ovi-, ovo-, gamete, ovum

egg-shaped: oviform, ovoid

egg yolk: vitellus

eighth cranial nerve: acoustic, vestibulocochlear

ejaculate: semen

ejaculation: ejection, emission, orgasm

ejaculation, slow: bradyspermatism

elasticity: resilience

elbow: humerus, radius, ulna joint, olecranon, cubitus; anconeal

elbow, below: subanconeus

elbow, in front of: antecubital

elbow, toward: anconad

elbow, tuberculosis of: olecranarthrocace

elbow diseases: anconagra, olecranarthropathy

elbow inflammation: anconitis, epicondylitis, olecranarthritis, olenitis

elbowlike: anconoid

elbow pain: epicondylalgia

electrical capacity unit: farad

electrical charge: action potential

electricity: faraday, galvanism

electricity, fear of: electrophobia

electric shock: electroconvulsive therapy

electrocardiographic recording: readout, tracing

electrolyte imbalance: hyperkalemia, hypernatremia, hypocalcemia, hypokalemia, hypomagnesemia, hyponatremia

electrolytes: bicarbonate, calcium, chloride, magnesium, phosphate, potassium, sodium, sulfate

Elephant man's disease: multiple neuroma, neurofibromatosis, neuromatosis, von Recklinghausen's disease

elevation: cumulus, eminence, mons, tubercle, tuberosity

elevator: levator

eleventh cranial nerve: accessory

elimination: cacation, defecation, dejecta, egesta, ejecta, enema, evacuate, excrement, excretion, sweat, urination, void

emaciation: anorexia, atrophy, cachexia, geromarasmus, inanition, malnutrition, marasmus, phthisis, skeletinization, starvation, symptosis

embryo: -blast, brepho-, blastocele, blastocyst, conceptus, ectoderm, entoderm, mesoderm, morola, trophoblast

embryo, extrauterine: eccyesis, ectopic pregnancy

embryo, membranes of: amnion, chorion

embryo destruction: abortion,
craniotomy, embryectomy,
embryoctony, embryotocia,
embryotomy
See also fetus destruction
embryo development: embryogenesis
embryo-like: embryoid, embryonoid
embryo stages: blastula, gastrula,
morula, zygote
emetics: apomorphine, ipecac
emigration: diapedesis, diapiresis,
migration, passage
eminence: agger, mons, projection,
prominence, tubercle
emotion: affect
emotion, lack of: apathy, athymic
emotion, release of: abreaction,
catharsis
emotional disturbance: affectomotor
emotionally dependent: anaclisis
emotionless: acathexis
emptiness, fear of: kenophobia
empty: deplete, void
empyema, gas with: pneumoempyema
encircle: cerclage
enclosed: encapsulated, encased,
enclave, insheathed, saccate
encompassing: ambient
end: tele-, apex, extremity
endbrain: telencephalon
endocrine disease: endocrinopathy,
pathocrinia
endocrine glands: pineal body,
pituitary, thyroid, parathyroid,
thymus, adrenal, pancreas, gonads
See also glands
endocrine specialist: endocrinologist
endometrium, extrinsic: endometriosis
endometrium disease: endometrioma
endometrium inflammation:
endometritis
endoscopes: arthroscope, bronchoscope,
colonoscope, colposcope,
duodenoscope, esophagoscope,
fetoscope, fiberscope, gastroscope,
hysteroscope, laparoscope,
laryngoscope, lithoscope,
observerscope, proctoscope,
sigmoidoscope

enema: clysma, clyster
energy, lack of: anergia, anergy,
asthenia
energy, mental: cathexis
energy production: anabolism
enhancer: synergist
enlargement: amplification, auxesis,
dilation, distention, expansion,
growth, hypertrophy,
intumescence, magnification,
swelling, tuber, tumefaction,
tumor, turgescence
entire: hol-, holo-
entrance: aditus, introitus, limen,
porta, threshold
environment: ambience, milieu
enzyme action: fermentation,
zymolysis
enzyme formation: zymogenesis
enzyme inhibitors: cilastatin,
poligeenan, sodium amylosulfate
enzymelike: zymoid
enzyme precursor: zymogen
enzymes: -ase, zymo-, acetolase,
adenase, adenosine hydrolase,
adenosine kinase, adenosine
triphosphatase, adenylate kinase,
aldolase, amidase, amidohydrolase,
aminoacylase, amylase, amylopsin,
asparaginase, aspartate kinase,
aspartate transaminase,
aspartoacylase, carbamate kinase,
carboxyhydrase, carboxylase,
carboxypeptidase, catalase,
cellulase, cholinesterase, chymase,
chymopapain, chymotrypsin,
coagulase, coenzyme A, creatinase,
cytochrome oxidase, deamidase,
deaminase, deoxyribonuclease,
dextrase, diastase, dipeptidase,
elastinase, endonuclease, enolase,
enterokinase, esterase, exonuclease,
fibrinase, fibrinogenase,
fructofuranosidase, galactosidase,
gelatinase, gluconolactonase,
histaminase, histozyme, hydrase,
hydratase, hydrolase, isocitrate
dehydrogenase, isoenzyme,
kallikrein, kinase, lactase, lactate

dehydrogenase, lactic
dehydrogenase, lactocidase,
lactolase, lipase, lysozyme, maltase,
muramidase, mutase, myokinase,
myosinase, nuclease, nucleosidase,
nucleotidase, oxidase, oxygenase,
pancreatin, pancrelipase, papain,
pectase, penicillinase, pepsin,
peptidase, peroxidase, phosphatase,
phosphodiesterase,
phosphohydrolase, phosphonuclease,
phosphoribosyl transferase,
phosphorylase, phytase, plasmin,
polynucleotidase, prolinase,
protease, proteinase,
prothrombinase, ptyalin, reductase,
renin, rennin, ribonuclease,
saccharase, staphylokinase,
steapsin, streptodornase,
streptokinase, sutilains, thrombin,
toxenzyme, transaminase,
transferase, triokinase, trypsin,
tyrosinase, urease, uricase, urico-
oxidase, urokinase, vesiculase,
zymase, zyme, zymose, zytase
enzymes, absence: anenzymia, azymia
enzymes, inactive: proenzyme,
proferment
enzymes, study of: enzymology
enzymes in urine: enzymuria
epidemic: plague
epidemic, widespread: pandemic
epididymis excision:
epididymodeferentectomy,
epididymo-orchidectomy,
epidymovasectomy
epididymis incision: epididymotomy
epididymis inflammation: epididymitis,
epididymo-orchitis
epididymis surgery:
epididymovasostomy
epididymis tumor: spermatocele,
spermatocyst
epigastrium hernia: epigastrocele
epigastrium pain: epigastralgia
epigastrium suturing:
epigastrorrhaphy

epiglottis excision: epiglottidectomy
epiglottis inflammation: epiglottiditis,
epiglottitis
epilepsy-like: epileptiform, epileptoid
epilepsy preventive: antiepileptic
epilepsy producing: epileptogenic
epileptic seizure: ictus
epileptic seizure, after: postictal
epinephrine activation: adrenergic
epinephrine in blood: adrenalinemia
epinephrine inhibition: adrenolytic
epinephrine in urine: adrenalinuria
epinephrine-related: adrenergic,
sympathomimetic
epithelioma: Jacob's ulcer,
Krompecher's tumor
epithelium-like: epitheloid
equal: iso-, peer
equilibrium: homeostasis
eradication: ablation
erection: distension, intumescence,
tumescence, turgescence
erection abnormalities: chordee,
impotence, mentulagra, Peyronie's
disease, priapism
erosion: abrasion, ulceration
eruption: blister, lesion, pox, pustule,
rash, wheal
eruption, in mouth: enanthema
erysipelas: phlogosis
erythrocyte: *See* red blood cell
esophagus dilation: esophagectasia
esophagus diseases: achalasia,
cardiospasm, reflux
esophagus examination:
esophagogastroscopy
esophagus excision: esophagectomy
esophagus hernia: esophagocele
esophagus incision: esophagotomy
esophagus inflammation: esophagitis,
periesophagitis
esophagus narrowing:
esophagostenosis, lemostenosis
esophagus pain: esophagalgia,
esophagodynia
esophagus paralysis: lemoparalysis

esophagus prolapse: esophagoptosis
esophagus softening: esophagomalacia
esophagus spasm: esophagismus,
    esophagospasm
esophagus surgery:
    esophagoenterostomy,
    esophagogastrostomy,
    esophagoplasty, esophagoplication,
    esophagostomy
estrogens: chlorotrianisene, dienestrol,
    diethylstilbestrol, equilin, estradiol,
    estriol, estrofurate, estrone,
    estropipate, ethinyl estradiol,
    fenestrel, mestranol, nylestriol,
    quinestrol
ether addiction: etheromania
etiology, unknown: agnogenic,
    idiopathic
eunuchlike: eunuchoid
eustachian tube: salping-, salpingo-,
    eustachium, salpinx, syrinx
eustachian tube discharge: tuborrhea
eustachian tube inflammation:
    eustachitis, salpingitis, syringitis
eustachian tube obstruction:
    salpingemphraxis,
    salpingostenochoria
evacuate: defecate, eject, eliminate,
    expel, urinate, void
eversion: ectropion
everything, fear of: panphobia
evident: patent, phanic
evisceration: exenteration
exaggerated reflexes: hyperreflexia
examination: -scopy, auscultation,
    biopsy, celioscopy, exploration,
    laparotomy, palpation, percussion.
    See also tests
examine: -scope
excess: ultra-, supernumerary
excessive: an-, ana-, hyper-, copious
excision: ablation, amputation, biopsy,
    extirpation, resection
excrement: scato-, egesta, ejecta, feces
excrement, fear of: coprophobia
excretion: dejecta, egesta, ejecta,
    feces, perspiration, sweat, urine

excretion, abnormal: allochezia,
    dyschezia
excretion, ammonia: ammonirrhea
excretion, diminished: hypoeccrisia
excretion, excessive: hypereccrisia
excretion promotor: eccritic
exercise: active, aerobic, dynamic,
    isokinetic, isometric, isotonic,
    passive, static
exercise treatment: kinesiatrics,
    kinesitherapy
exertion, lack of: aponia
exhaustion: asthenia, burnout,
    enervation, inanition, prostation
exhaustion, nervous: neurasthenia
existing, sense of: cenesthesia
exocrine glands: lacrimal, mammary,
    salivary, sebaceous, sweat
expanding: velamentous
expansion: amplification, dilation,
    enlargement, magnification,
    rarefaction
expectant: gravid, pregnant
expectorants: bromhexine,
    guaifenesin, terpin hydrate
experience: empiric
exposure: hypothermia
exposure of genitals: exhibitionism
expulsion: discharge, ejaculation,
    evacuation, excretion, voiding
expulsion promoter: -agog, -agogue
extension backward: dorsiflexion
extensive: comprehensive, in-depth,
    vastus
external: ecto-, exo-, extra-, extro-
extirpation: ablation
extremities, fusion: sirenomelia,
    symmelia, sympus, tripodia
extremity: acro-, mel-, melo-, acral,
    ankle, arm, digits, fingers, foot,
    forearm, hand, hip, leg, limbs,
    shoulder, thigh, toes, wrist
extremity, artificial: prosthesis
extremity, fall asleep: temporary
    hypesthesia
extremity, large: acromegaly,
    megalomelia

extremity, premature aging of:
acrogeria
extremity, small: acromicria
extremity amputation: dismember
extremity disorders: acroarthritis,
acroasphyxia, acroataxia,
acrocinesia, acrocyanosis,
acrodermatitis, acrocontracture,
acrohypothermy, acrokinesia,
acrometagenesis, acromyotonia,
acroneurosis, acroparesthesia,
acropathy, acroscleroderma,
acrotrophoneurosia, ectromelia,
erythromelalgia, hemimelia,
phocomelia, Raynaud's sign,
rodonalgia
extremity edema: acroedema
extremity numbness: obdormition
extremity pain: acroesthesia
extremity paralysis: quadraplegia
eye: oculo-, ophthalm-, ophthalmo-,
optico-, opto-, canthus, choroid,
conjunctiva, cornea, iris, lens,
ocular, oculus, ophthalmus,
pterygium, pupil, retina, sclera
See also blindness, color blindness,
vision
eye, abnormal vision: ametropia,
anisometropia, astigmatism,
hemianopsia, hypermetropia,
hyperopia, myopia, platymorphia,
presbyopia, quadrantanopsia,
scieropia, scotodinia, scotoma,
tetartanopia, tetartanopsia,
triplopia
eye, absence: anophthalmos, anopia
eye, around: circumorbital
eye, bands in: angioid streaks
eye, behind: retrobulbar, retro-ocular
eye, bleeding: Eales' disease, hyphema,
ophthalmorrhagia, ophthalmorrhea
eye, colorless: aniridia
eye, farsighted: hypermetropia,
hyperopia
eye, large: megalophthalmus
eye, light flashes in: scintillation,
synchysis

eye, nearsighted: brachymetropia,
myopia
eye, near vision improvement:
gerontopia, senopia
eye, normal: emmetropia
eye, pressure in: buphthalmos,
glaucoma, hydrophthalmos
eye, pupil contraction: miosis
eye, pus in: pyophthalmia,
pyophthalmitis
eye, small: microphthalmos,
nanophthalmos
eye, spots before: floaters, muscae
volitantes, vitreous floaters
eye, science of: ophthalmology
eye abnormalities: corectopia,
cryptophthalmus, cyclopia,
enophthalmos, entropion,
synophthalmia, synopsia,
triplokoria
eye adhesions: syncanthus, synechia
eye adjustment: accommodation,
isometropia, photopia, scotopia
eyeball: bulbar, orb, vitreous humor
eyeball, large: macrophthalmia
eyeball atrophy: ophthalmatrophy,
phthisis bulbi
eyeball prolapse: enophthalmos,
proptosis
eyeball rupture: ophthalmorrhexis
eyeball socket: orbit
eyebrow: supercilium
eyebrow, loss of: anaphalantiasis,
madarosis, milphosis
eyebrow fusion: synophrys
eyebrows, between: glabella,
intercilium, mesophyron
eyebrows, thick: hypertrichophrydia
eye constrictor: miotic
eye deviation: adtorsion, anaphoria,
anatropia, anoopsia, anophoria,
anopsia, anotropia, catatropia,
conclination, cyclophoria,
cyclotropia, esophoria, esotropia,
exocataphoria, exophoria,
heterophoria, heterotropia,
hyperphoria, hypoesophoria,
hypoexophoria, hypophoria,

incyclotropia, katophoria, katotropia, periphoria, strabismus, tropia, vergence

eye deviation, downward: hypotropia

eye deviation, inward: esophoria, esotropia

eye deviation, outward: exotropia

eye deviation, upward: hypertropia

eye dilator: atropine, mydriatic

eye diseases: aeluropsis, ametropia, aniseikonia, anisocoria, anisometropia, antimetropia, arcus juvenilis, arcus senilia, astigmatism, cataract, chorioretinopathy, choroideremia, coloboma, detached retina, Duane's syndrome, embryotoxon, fibroplasia, Foville's paralysis, gonorrheal ophthalmia, hypocyclosis, hypopyon, hysteropia, iridodonesis, Irving-Gass syndrome, megalopsia, micropsia, oculopathy, onyx, ophthalmoblennorrhea, ophthalmopathy, photoretinitis, presbyopia, pseudoglioma, pterygium, retrolental, scintillating scotoma, sclerophthalmia, spintherism, teichopsia, teleopsia, tunnel vision, xanthopsia, xerophthalmia

eye doctor: ophthalmologist, oculist; optometrist

eye edema: chemosis, papilledema

eye examinations: angiography, belonoskiascopy, chromoscopy, electoretinogram, fluorescein, goncoscopy, ophthalmoscopy, reclination, retinoscopy, skiascopy, tonography, tonometry
See also eye tests

eye exercises: orthoptics, pleoptics

eye fluid: aqueous humor

eyeglasses: bifocal, contact lenses, corrective lenses, trifocal, spectacles, undine

eyeground: fundus

eye growth: drusen, encanthis

eye infection: mycophthalmia, oculomycosis, ophthalmomycosis

eye inflammation: canaliculitis, chalkitis, chorioretinitis, choroiditis, choroidocyclitis, choroidoiritis, choroidoretinitis, conjunctivitis, cyclitis, cyclochoroiditis, dacryocystitis, endophthalmitis, episcleritis, hyalitis, ophthalmia, ophthalmitis, ophthalmodesmitis, ophthalmomyitis, ophthalmoneuritis, panophthalmia, papillitis, parophthalmia, periphacitis, photophthalmia, scleritis, sclerochoroiditis, scleroconjunctivitis, scleroiritis, sclerokeratitis, sclerokeratoiritis, trachoma, uveitis, xenophthalmia

eye instruments: anaclasimeter, biomicroscope, electroretinograph, gonioscope, oculometroscope, ophthalmoscope, perimeter, slit lamp, tonometer

eyelash: blephar-, blepharo-, cili-, cilia

eyelash, abnormal: entropion, trichiasis, tristichia

eyelash disorder: distichiasis, polystichia

eyelash excision: ciliectomy

eyelash formation: ciliogenesis

eyelash loss: deplumation, madarosis, milphosis, ptilosis

eyelash surgery: ciliarotomy

eye lens, lack of: aphakia

eye lens removal: extraction

eyelid: blephar-, blepharo-, cili-, cilia, palpebra

eyelid, abnormal: blepharelosis, ectropion, entropion

eyelid, absence: ablepharia

eyelid, large: macroblepharia

eyelid, small: microblepharon

eyelid adhesion: ankyloblepharon, blepharosynechia, symblepharon

eyelid cartilage, softening:
    tarsomalacia
eyelid discharge: blepharopyorrhea,
    blepharorrhea
eyelid diseases: blepharocoloboma,
    lagophthalmos, pladaroma,
    pseudoptosis, schizoblepharia,
    xanthelasma
eyelid droop: blepharochalasis,
    blepharoplegia, blepharoptosis,
    Horner's syndrome, ptosis
eyelid edema: blepharedema,
    varicoblepharon
eyelid edge: tarso-
eyelid excision: blepharectomy,
    blepharosphincterectomy
eyelid hardening: scleriasis
eyelid incision: blepharotomy
eyelid inflammation: blepharadenitis,
    blepharitis, blepharoadenitis,
    blepharoconjunctivitis,
    endophthalmitis, psorophthalmia,
    tarsadenitis, tarsitis
eyelid muscle spasm: blepharospasm
eyelid paralysis: blepharoplegia
eyelid plastic surgery: blepharoplasty,
    tarsocheiloplasty, tarsoplasty
eyelid retraction: paraphimosis oculi
eyelids, between: interpalpebral
eyelids, slit between: canthus
eyelid separation, excessive:
    blepharodiastasis
eyelid slit narrowed: blepharophimosis,
    blepharostenosis
eyelid spasm: blepharoclonus,
    blepharospasm, cillosis, nictitating
    spasm
eyelid surgery: blepharorrhaphy,
    cyclectomy, cyclicotomy,
    tarsectomy, tarsorrhaphy,
    tarsotomy
eyelid thickened: blepharopachynsis,
    pachyblepharon
eyelid tumors: blepharoadenoma,
    blepharoatheroma, blepharoncus,
    blepharophyma, chalazion,
    encanthis, meibomian cyst,
    tarsophyma

eyelid twitching: blepharism
eye membranes: choroid, ciliary body
eye movement: microstrabismus,
    nystagmus, oculogyration,
    oculomotor, ophthalmogyric,
    opsoclonus, saccade, vergence
eye ointment: oculentum
eye pain: hereropharalgia,
    ophthalmagra, ophthalmalgia,
    ophthalmodynia, photalgia
eye paralysis: ophthalmoplegia
eyepiece: ocular
eye position, normal: mesoropter
eye protrusion: choriocele,
    exophthalmos, ophthalmocele,
    ophthalmoptosis, sclerectasia
eye pupil contraction agent: miotic
eye refraction measurement:
    pupilloscopy, retinoscopy, skiascopy
eye removal: enucleation, exenteration
eyes, around: circumocular,
    circumorbital, periocular,
    periorbital
eyes, between: interorbital
eyes, fear of: ommatophobia
eye skin folds: epicanthus
eye softening: ophthalmomalacia,
    ophthalmophthisis
eye spasm: ophryosis, ophthalmospasm
eye spot: scotoma
eyestrain: asthenopia, ophthalmocopia
eye surgery: corelysis, couching,
    evisceroneurotomy, excision,
    keratoleptynsis, ophthalmectomy,
    ophthalmomyotomy,
    ophthalmophlebotomy,
    ophthalmoplasty, orbitomy,
    peritomy, radial keratotomy,
    reclination, rhinocanthectomy,
    rhinommectomy,
    sclerectoiridectomy, sclerectomy,
    scleroplasty, sclerostomy,
    sclerotomy, tenomyotomy,
    uveoplasty
eye tests: Amsler grid, Bjerrum's
    screen, Holmgren's, hyaluronidase,
    Jaeger's, Nagel's, Snellen's

eyetooth: canine
eye tumor: glioma
eye variation: dextrocularity, sinistrocular
eyewash: collyrium
eye weakness: asthenopia
eye white: sclera

F

face: facio-, prospo-, forehead, eyes, nose, cheeks, lips, jaw; countenance, physiognomy, visage
face, absent: aprosopia
face, broad: platyopia
face, diagnosis from: physiognosis
face, large: megaprosopous, prosopectasia
face, lines in: prosopoanoschisis
face abnormality: ateloprosopia, prosopus varus
face bandage: accipiter
face cleft: macrostomia, prosoposchisis, schistoprosopia, schizoprosopia
face downward: pronation
face lift: cosmetic surgery, facioplasty, plastic surgery, rhinoplasty, rhytidectomy
face muscle: pterygoid, temporal, zygomatic
face pain: erythroprosopalgia, opsialgia
face paralysis: Bell's palsy, facioplegia, prosopoplegia
face plastic surgery: chalinoplasty, mentoplasty, rhinoplasty
face presentation: prosopotocia
faces, inability to recognize: prosopagnosia
face spasm: Chvostek's sign, prosopospasm, risus sardonicus
face upward: supination
failure, fear of: kakorrhaphiophobia
faintness: lipothymia, lipsis animi, syncope, unconsciousness

fake treatment: placebo
fall: descensus
fall asleep, of extremity: temporary hypesthesia
fall forward: prevertiginous
falling: descensus, prolapse, ptosis
falling off: deciduous, deterioration
falling sickness: epilepsy
fallopian tube: salping-, salpingo, salpinx
fallopian tube, blood in: hematosalpinx
fallopian tube, pus in: pyosalpinx
fallopian tube disease: hematosalpinx, pyrosalpinx
fallopian tube distension: hydroparasalpinx, hydrosalpinx, sactosalpinx
fallopian tube fixation: adnexopexy, salpingopexy
fallopian tube hernia: salpingocele, salpingo-oophorocele, salpingo-oothecocele
fallopian tube inflammation: endosalpingitis, myosalpingitis, perisalpingitis, pyrosalpingitis, salpingitis, salpingo-oophoritis, salpingo-oothecitis, salpingoperitonitis
fallopian tube surgery: acrohysterosalpingectomy, celiosalpingectomy, fallectomy, fallostomy, salpingectomy, salpingo-oophorectomy, salpingo-ovariectomy, salpingorrhaphy, salpingosalpingostomy, salpingostomatomy, salpingostomy, salpingotomy, salpingoureterostomy
fall out: defluvium
false: pseudo-
false labor: Braxton-Hicks contraction
false teeth: bridge, denture, plate
fang: tooth
fantasy state: delusion, dereism
farmer's lung: hypersensitivity alveolitis

far off: tel-, tele-
far-sighted: hypermetropia, hyperopia
farther: ultra-
fascia inflammation: fasciitis
fascia surgery: fasciectomy,
  fasciodesis, fascioplasty,
  fasciorrhaphy
fastening: fixation
fasting: abrosia
fat: adip-, adipo-, lip-, lipo-, pimel-,
  stearo-, stearo-, steato-, dipose,
  corpulent, endomorphic,
  hyperadiposis, lipid, lipoid, obese,
  pimelosis, sebum, steatorrhea,
  triglycerides, ventricose
  fat, excess:
  adiposity, hyperlipemia,
  hyperlipoproteinemia, hyperliposis,
  lipacidemia, lipaciduria, lipomatosis
fat, hernia: adipocele, liparocele
fat, lack of: hypoliposis
fat accumulation: adipopexia, adiposis,
  bitrochanteric, lipodystrophy,
  lipopexia, liposis
fatal: lethal, malignant, pernicious,
  toxic, virulent
fat cell: lipocyte
fat cell, immature: lipoblast
fat cell destruction: adiponecrosis
fat cell tumor: Abernathy's sarcoma,
  liposarcoma
fat conversion: adipolysis, lipoclasis,
  lipodieresis, lipolysis, lipophagic,
  saponification, steatolysis
fat deposits in arteries: arteriosclerosis,
  atherogenesis, atheroma,
  atherosclerosis
fat deposits in buttocks: steatopygia
fat disorders: adipocele, Dercum's,
  lipidosis, lipocele, lipodystrophy,
  lipomatosis, lipopexia
fat formation: adipogenesis,
  lipogenesis
fat-free: defatted
fatigue: apocamnosis
fatigue, disease related: adynamia,
  asthenia

fatigue, extreme: exhaustion
fatigue, fear of: kopophobia
fat in blood: lipemia, pionemia
fat in urine: adiposuria, lipuria,
  pimeluria
fatlike: adipoid, lipoid, steariform
fat metabolism disorders:
  abetalipoproteinemia, Weber-
  Christian disease
fat removal: adipectomy, lipectomy
fat tissue degeneration: steatosis
fat tissue destruction: adiponecrosis,
  steatonecrosis
fat tissue inflammation: lipoarthritis,
  lipogranuloma, panniculitis,
  pimelitis, steatitis
fat tumor: adipoma, liparocele,
  lipochondroma, lipofibroma, lipoma,
  liposarcoma, pimeloma, steatoma
fatty: steato-, sebaceous
fatty stool: pimelorrhea, steatorrhea
fauces inflammation: faucitis
fauces paralysis: isthmoparalysis,
  isthmoplegia
fault: defect, flaw, imperfection,
  vitium
fear: anxiety, fright, phobia,
  polyphobia
  See also phobias
fear, generalized: panophobia,
  panphobia, pantophobia
fearing, fear of: phobophobia
feathers, fear of: pteronophobia
feathers, having: -pennet
feather-shaped: bipenniform,
  multipenniform, penniform
feathery growth: plumose
febrile stage: intrafebrile, intrapyretic
feces: copr-, copro-, scato-, sterco-,
  dejecta, egesta, excrement,
  excreta, ordure, stercus, stool
feces, abnormal interest in: coprophilia
feces, eroticism from: coprolagnia
feces, fat in: pimelorrhea, steatorrhea
feces, fear of: coprophobia,
  rhypophobia, scatophobia

feces, hard: copralith, fecalith, fecaloma, scatoma, scybalum, stercolith, stercoroma
feces, incontinent: copracrasis, encopresis, scatacratia, scoracratia
feces, pus in: pyochezia, pyofecia
feces, study of: coprology, scatology
feces, vomiting: copremesis
feces eating: coprophagy, rhypophagy, scatophagy
feces examination: scatoscopy
feces excretion, abnormal: allochezia, dyschezia
feceslike: stercorous
feces of newborn: meconium
feebleminded: mental retardation, oligergasia
feeding on: -varous, saprophyte
feedings: breast, gastrogavage, gastrostomy, gavage, intravenous, parenteral nutrition
feeling: -aesthesia, -esthesia, affect, esthesia
feeling, loss of: anesthesia
feelings, expressed: abreaction, acting out, catharsis
feet: *See* foot
female: gyn-, gyne-, gyneco-, gyno-, girl, woman
female inheritance: hologynic
female sex organs: clitoris, mons, labia majora, labia minora, vagina, vervix, uterus, fallopian tubes, ovary
female sex organs, examination: culdoscopy
female trouble: gynecologic problems, hysterectomy
femur hernia: merocele
femur process: bitrochanter, trochanter
ferment: enzyme
fermentation: zymolsis, zymosis
fermentation preventive: antifermentative, antizymotic
fertile: fecundity, fruitful, progenerative, prolific, reproductive, uberous, virile

fertilization: conception, fecundation, gametes, impregnation, insemination, reproduction, saturation, semination, syngamy
fertilization, multiple: hypercyesia, multifetation, superfecundation, superfetation, superimpregnation
fester: abscess, necrose, putrefy, putresce, suppurate, ulcerate
fetal blood vessels: ductus arteriosus
fetal distress: asphyxia, hypoxia
fetal membrane, rupture: amniorrhexis
fetal membranes: allantois, amnion, chorion
fetal movement: quickening
fetal tumor: oncofetal
fetus: brepho-, embryo
fetus, measurement of: fetometry
fetus, ossified: lithopedion, ostembryon, osteopedion, papyraceus
fetus, study of: fetology, embryology
fetus, turning: version
fetus covering: vernix caseosa
fetus deformed, causing: teratogen, teratogenesis
fetus deformed, fear of: teratophobia
fetus deformed, study of: teratology
fetus deformed, twins: anadidymus, triophthalmos, triopodymus
See also twins, conjoined
fetus examination: fetography, fetoscopy
fetus fluid: amniotic
fetus malformed: terato-, augnathus, cephalomelus, cryptocephalus, cyclopia, derodidymus, dicephalus, opocephalus, opodiymus, synophthalmia, teras, teratosis, triocephalus, triophthalmos, triopodymus
fetus measurement: fetometry
fetus nutrition: embryotrophy
fetus surgery: cephalotomy, cleidotomy, embryotomy, encephalotomy, excerebration

fever: pyr-, pyret-, pyreto-, typho-, ague, calentura, febres, febrile, pyrexia
fever, after: metapyretic, postpyretic
fever, artificial treatment: pyretherapy, pyretotherapy
fever, before: antefebrile, antepyretic
fever, caused by: pyreticosis
fever, fear of: fibriphobia, pyrexeophobia
fever, lack of: afebrile, apyretic, apyrexia
fever, malarial: ague
fever blister: cold sore, Herpes simplex
fever increase: fervescence
fever origin: pyretogenesia
fever producing: febrifacient, hyperpyrexia, hyperthermia, physiocopyrexia, pyretogen, pyretogenic, pyrexin
fever reducer: alexipyretic, algefacient, antifebrile, antipyretic, antithermic, febricide, febrifuge, refrigerant
fever reduction: lysis, pyretolysis
few: olig-, oligo-
fiber: cellulose
fibrillation, stopping: cardioversion, defibrillation
fibrin, excess: fibrinosis
fibrin, lack of: hypinosis, hypoinosemia
fibrin in urine: fibrinuria
fibrin(ogen) deficiency: afibrinogenemia, fibrinopenia, hypofibrinogenemia
fibroids: leiomyoma uteri
fibroid tumor surgery: fibroidectomy, fibromectomy
fibrous tissue development: fibroplasia, fibrosis
fibrous tissue formation: fibrosis
fibrous tissue inflammation: fibrositis, initis, inochondritis, inositis, myositis, tendonitis
fibula: peroneo-, peroneal

fifth cranial nerve: trigeminal
fifth day: quintan
fifth disease: erythema infectiosum
file: raspatory, xyster
fill: pack
filtering: colation
filth, eating of: rhypophagy, scatophagy
filth, fear of: automysophobia, mysophobia, rhypophobia, rupophobia
final: definitive
finger: dactyl-, dactylo-, dactyldigit, digital, phalange
    See also digits, extremities, toe
finger diseases: acro-osteolysis, acroscleroderma, sclerodactylia, xyrospasm
finger fusion: palmature
finger infection: felon, whitlow
finger joint: knuckle
fingernail: *See* nail
fingerprints: dactylogram, dermatoglyphics
fingerprints, examination: dactyloscopy
fingerprints, study of: dactylography
fingers, abnormal: clinodactyly
fire: pyro-, erysipelas, ignis
fire, fear of: pyrophobia
fire, love of: pyrolagnia, pyromania
firm: scleroid
first: arch-, arche-, archi-, proto-, princeps, protal
first case: index case, proband, propositus
first cranial nerve: olfactory
fish, fear of: ichthyophobia
fish poisoning: ichthyosarcotoxism
fishskin disease: ichthyosis
fission reproduction: schizogenesis
fissure: cleft, cleavage, crevice, diastoma, division, groove, interstice, rhagadeform, rhagades, rima, rimose, scissura, split, sulcus
fissure, abdominal: schistocelia
fissure, eyelid: schizoblepharia

fissure, face: schistoprosopia, schizoprosopia
fissure, thorax: schistothorax
fistula: syrinx
fit: convulsion, ictus, seizure
fitted together: apposition, contiguity, juxtaposition
fixation: -pexy, anchorage, attachment, delusion, monomania, obsession
fixed: ankylosed, spayed, stabile
flabby: flaccid, pulpy, pultaceous
flake: lepido-
flank: ilium latus
flap: cusp
flapping: asterixis
flapping tremor: asterixis
flare: erythema
flask: retort
flask-shaped: lageniform
flat: plano-, facet, plane, planum
flatfoot: pes planovalgus, pes planus, talipes valgus
flatfooted: platypodia, sarapus
flatness: nonresonance, applanation
flatulence, noise from: borborygmus, crepitus
flatworms: cestodes, trematodes
    See also flukes, tapeworms
flaw: defect, disfigurement, scar
flea: Pulex
flea destruction: depulization, pulicide
flea infested: publicatio
flesh: sarco-
    See also skin, soft tissue
flesh, hard: neonatorum scirrhosarca, sclerema
flesh breakdown: sarcolysis
flesh eating: carnivorous, sarcophagy
fleshlike: carnose, sarcoid
flesh producing: sarcogenic, sarcopoietic, sarcotic
flesh tumor: sarcoadenoma, sarcocarcinoma, sarcocele, sarcoid, sarcomphalocele, sarcomyces, sarcosis

fleshy: carneous
fleshy growth: carnosity, caruncle
flexible: adaptable, pliant, resilient, supple, tensile
flint disease: chalicosis
floaters: muscae volitantes
floods, fear of: antlophobia
flow: -rhea, rheo-
flow, excessive: flux, profluvium
flow back: reflux, regurgitation
flowers, fear of: anthophobia
flowing out: effluent, flux
flu: influenza
fluctuation: ambivalence, oscillation
fluid, across membrane: transudation
fluid, desire for: thirst
fluid, excessive secretion: polyrrhea
fluid accumulation: anasarca, congestion, edema
fluid-cell imbalance: hydremia
fluid in abdomen: ascites, hydroperitoneum
fluid in body cavity: effusion
fluid in ear: hydrotis, hydrotympanum
fluid injector: syringe
fluid in peritoneum: ascites, hydroperitoneum, seroperitoneum
fluid in pleural cavity: hydrothorax
fluid intake: -posia, drink
fluid in testes: hydrocele, hydrosarcocele
fluid loss: dehydration, extravasation
fluid removal: aspiration, dehydration, paracentesis, tapping
fluids: blood, decoction, extracellular, exudate, fluidextract, infusion, interstitial, intracellular, lacrimal, liniment, lymph, mucus, oleoresin, plasma, saliva, semen, seminal, serum, succus, synovia, tincture, urine
    See also liquid, water
fluids, in equilibrium, science of: hydrostatics
fluids injected under skin: hypodermoclysis

fluids in motion, science of:
  hydrokinetics
fluids into body: clysis, infuse, inject
fluid storage: reservoir
fluke diseases: echinostomiasis,
  fascioliasis, fasciolopsiasis, halzoun,
  heterophydiasis, opisthorchiasis,
  schistosomiasis, trematodiasis
flukes: Clonorchis, Fascioloides,
  Fasciolopsis, Gastrodiscoides,
  Heterophyes, Metagonimus,
  Opisthorchis, Paragonimus,
  Schistosoma, trematodes
  See also liver flukes
flutter: fremitus, palpitation
fly: Musca
fly, Spanish: cantharides
fog, fear of: homichlophobia
fold: convolution, flexure, fornix,
  frenulum, plica, plication,
  reduplication, ruga
fondle: contrectation
food: troph-, tropho-, aliment,
  nutriment, nourishment
food, fear of: sitophobia
food, inability to chew: amasesis
food, lack of craving: inappetence
food allergy: hypersensitivity reaction
food aversion: anorexia, apositia,
  asitia, cibophobia, fastidium
food ball: phytobezoar
food breakdown: catabolism, digestion
food conversion: chylosis
food craving: bulimia, opsomania,
  oreximania, phagomania,
  sitomania
food depravation: abrosia, starvation
food poisoning: botulism
food therapy: hyperalimentation,
  parenteral nutrition, sitotherapy,
  superalimentation, suralimentation
foolhardiness: hyperthymia
foolishness: moria
foot: pedi-, pod-, podo-, extremity,
  pedal, pes, planta, sole
foot, abnormal: atelopodia, cavus,
  Morton's disease, Morton's foot,
  Morton's neuralgia, Morton's toe,
  polyphalangism, polypodia, talipes

foot, absence: apodal, apodia, apus
foot, athlete's: ringworm infection
foot, excessive sweating:
  acrohyperhidrosis
foot, instep: tarso-
foot, large: macropodia, pachypodous,
  pes gigas
foot, small: micropodia
foot, study of: chiropody, podiatry,
  podology, sciopody
foot amputation: Syme's operation,
  Tripier's operation
foot anatomy: calcaneus, talus, cuboid,
  navicular cuneiform, metatarsals,
  phalanges, instep
foot bath: pediluvium
foot care: pedicure
foot deformities: pes cavus, talipes
foot diseases: athlete's foot, bunion,
  cryptopodia, dermatophytosis, ring
  worm, tinea pedis
foot extensor: plantarflexion
foot inflammation: podarthritis
footlike: pediculus, pediform
foot muscle: soleus
foot odor: podobromidrosis
foot pain: metatarsalgia, pedialgia,
  pedionalgia, podalgia, pododynia,
  tarsalfia
footprint: dermatoglyphics,
  ichnogram, pedograph
foot specialist: chiropodist, podiatrist
foot surgery: sphyrectomy,
  sphyrotomy, tarsotomy
foot treatment: chiropody
force: potency
force, backward: retrusion
force, inward: retrude
forceps: Adson, alligator, Allis, artery,
  Arruga, aural, Barton, Blaydes,
  Brown-Adson, bulldog, bullet,
  capsule, Chamberlen, clamp,
  Clayman, clip, Colibri, dental,
  dressing, Elliot, Evans, Fechner,
  Garrison, Goedman, Graefe,
  hemostatic, Hodge's, Hoffer-
  McPherson, Kazanjian, Kelly,
  Kelman-McPherson, Kjelland,
  Knapp's, Kocher, Lahey, Laplace,

McIndoe, McKenzie, McPherson,
Moore, mosquito, Neyvas, obstetric,
O'Hara, Parelman, Piper, Riegel,
Shepard, Storz, Tarnier, torsion,
Willett

forearm: antebrachium, antibrachium, cubitus, ulna and radius, upper extremity

forebrain: prosencephalon

forefinger: index finger

foregut: protogaster

forehead: frons, metopic

foreign: allotrio-, xeno-

foreign body, inflammation: perialienitis, perixenitis

foreskin: frenulum, glans penis, prepuce, preputium

foreskin, lack of: apellous, circumcised

foreskin inflammation: acrobystitis, acroposthitis, posthitis

foreskin removal: circumcision, posthetomy

foreskin surgery: posthioplasty

forest, fear of: hylophobia, ylophobia

forgetfulness: amnesia

forgetfulness, lack of: alethia

forked: bifurcation, furcal

form: spectro-, morphology, skeleton, template

formless: amorphous, anidean

forward: proso-

foul: nauseous, putrid, rancid

foul stomach: saburra

foundation: basi-, basio-

four-footed: quadruped

fourth cranial nerve: trochlear

fourth day: quartan

foxglove: digitalis

fracture: -clasis, break, diaclasia, fissured, greenstick, rhegma, syntripsis, thrypsis, tuft

fragment: clasmatosis, crumble, section, segment, specimen

framework: skeleton

fraternal twins: dizygotic twins

freckle: dermatocelidosis, dermatokelidosis, ephelis, lentigo, macula, tache

freeze-drying: lyophilization

freezing tissue: cryocautery, cryosurgery, hypothermia

frequency: pitch

frequent occurrence: endemic

Freudian stages: anal, genital, oral

friction, dry: ectrimma, xerotripsis

friction treatment: iatraliptic

fringe: fimbria

frogs, fear of: batrachophobia

from: ab-, abs-, de-

front: antero-, anterior, ventral

frontward: frontal, ventral

frontward movement: anterograde

frostbite: chilblain, congelation, kibe, pernio

frost itch: hiemalis, pruritus

frozen shoulder: adhesive capsulitis

fructose: levulose

fructose in blood: fructosemia, levulosemia

fructose in urine: fructosuria, levulosuria

fruit-eating: frugivorous

fruitful: fecund, uberous

full: -ulent, replete, satiety, saturated

functioning, fear of: ergasiophobia

fungus: myc-, myceto-, myco-, Acremonium, Aspergillus, Blastomyces, Candida, Coccidioides, Cryptococcus, epidermophyton, Fusarium, Geotrichum, Hemispara, Histoplasma, Mucor, Neurospora, Octomyces, Paracoccidiodes, Penicillium, Phycomycetes, Rhinosporidium, Saccharomyces, Sporothrix, Trichophyton, Trichosporon, yeasts, Zygomycetes

fungus, caused by: mycetogenic

fungus, induced by: mycetogenetic

fungus, study of: mycology

fungus disease: acremoniosis, aspergillosis, blastomycosis, candidiasis, chromomycosis, coccidioidomycosis, cryptococcosis, dermatomycosis, epidermophytosis, ergotism, favus, fungemia, geotrichosis, histoplasmosis, lobomycosis, mucormycosis, mycetoma, mycomyringitis,

mycophthalmia, mycosis, mycotica,
myringomycosis, otitis, otomycosis,
phycomycosis, piedra, rhinomycosis,
ringworm, saccharomycosis,
sporotrichosis, tinea barbae, tinea
capitis, tinea carporis, tinea
unquium, trichophytosis,
trichosporosis, zygomycosis
fungus growth, inhibited: fungistatic
fungus in blood: fungemia,
mycethemia, mycohemia
fungus killer: fungicide
funguslike: fungoid, mycoid
fungus poisoning: mycetism
fungus preventive: antifungal,
antimycotic
fungus therapy: *See* antifungals
funnel chest: chonechondrosternum,
pectus excavatum
funnel-shaped: choanoid,
infundibuliform
funnel-shaped opening: choana
funny bone: internal condyle of
humerus
fur, fear of: doraphobia
furrow: groove, sulcus
furrow, multiple: trisulcate
fuse: coalesce
fused: accretio, coalescence
fusiform-shaped: spindle
fusion: ankylosis, symphysis,
syzygium, syzygy
fusion malformation: synactosis

G

gag: asphyxiate, choke, convulse, gasp,
retch, suffocate
gag reflex: pharyngeal reflex
gaiety, fear of: cherophobia
gait, abnormal: brachybasia
galactose in urine: galactosuria
galactose in urine, lack of:
agalactosuria
gall: bili-, chol-, chole-, cholo-, bile

gallbladder: cholecyst
See also bile
gallbladder, pus in:
pyopneumocholecystitis
gallbladder calculus: cholecystolithiasis
gallbladder dilation: cholecystectasia
gallbladder displacement:
cholecystoptosis
gallbladder disease: cholecystopathy
gallbladder edema: hydrocholecystis
gallbladder examination:
cholecystography
gallbladder excision: cholecystectomy,
cystectomy
gallbladder incision:
cholecystocolotomy, cholecystotomy,
cystotomy
gallbladder inflammation: cholecystitis,
pericholecystitis
gallbladder pain: cholecystalgia
gallbladder surgery:
cholecystenterostomy,
cholecystnephrostomy,
cholecystocolostomy,
cholecystoduodenostomy,
cholecystogastrostomy,
cholecystoileostomy,
cholecystojejunostomy,
cholecystolithotomy,
cholecystostomy, cholelithotomy,
cystocalostomy, cystostomy
gallbladder suturing:
cholecystenterorrhaphy,
cholecystopexy, cholecystorrhaphy
gallsickness: anaplasmosis
gallstone: biliary calculus, calculus,
cholelithiasis, chololith
gallstone crushing:
cholecystolithotripsy
gallstone removal:
choledocholithotomy, cholelithotomy
gamma globulin, absence:
agammaglobulinemia,
hypogammaglobulinemia
ganglion inflammation: ganglionitis,
perigangliitis

gangrene: anthraconecrosis, Reynaud's disease, sphaceloderma
gangrenous: sphacelate
gaping: oscitation
gargoylism: Hurler's syndrome
gas: aero-, physo-, pneum-, pneumato-, pneumo-, flatulence, pneumatic, vapor
gas, distention: meteorism, physocele, physohematometra, physohydrometra, physometra, physopyosalpinx, tympanism
gas, intestinal: flatus, tympanites
gas, laughing: nitrous oxide
gas bacillus: Clostridium perfringens
gas bubbles in lung: decompression sickness
gaseous: aeriform
gaseous state: steam, vapor
gases: acetyline, air, butane, carbon dioxide, carbon monoxide, ether, helium, hydrogen, methane, nitrogen, nitrous oxide, oxygen, ozone, propane
gases, science of: pneumatology
gas exchange: respiration
gas gangrene: anaerobic myositis
gas in cranium: pneumocephalus, pneumoencephalus
gasp: rale, wheeze
gas production: aerogenesis
gas reducer: antiflatulent, carminative
gas therapy: carminative
gastric: *See* abdomen, stomach
gastric juice, excessive: gastrorrhea, gastrosuccorrhea, hyperchylia, polygastria
gastric juice, lack of: achylia, hypochylia, oligochylia
gastrointestinal tract: alimentary tract, digestive tract
gay: homosexual
gelling: stiffness
gender: female, male, sex
gene: allele
gene, inactive: amorph

gene change: halmatogenesis, mutagenesis, mutation, saltatory variation
generate: genesis
genetic terms: accessory chromosome, acquired, allele, anaphase, anastral, androgenesis, aneuploidy, aster, autodiploidy, autosome, banding, Barr bodies, centriole, centromere, chromatid, chromatin, chromosome, clevage, clone, codon, crossing over, deme, Denver classification, diploid, DNA, dominance, double helix, duplication, euploidy, gamete, gene, gene splicing, genetic code, genetic colonization, genetic counseling, genetic death, genetic drift, genetic engineering, genetic equilibrium, genetic isolate, genetic map, genetic marker, genetic screening, genotype, haploid, heterogamete, heterozygous, homogamete, homologous, homozygous, hybrid, hypostatic, inbreeding, inheritance, interphase , inversion, isogamete, isogeneic, karyotype, lethals, linkage, locus, mapping, marker gene, meiosis, Mendalism, metaphase, mitochondria, mitosis, monosome, mosaic, mutagen, mutation, nondisjunction, oncogene, ookinesis, operon, pedigree, phenotype, plasmagene, plasmotomy, prophase, recessive, recombination, replication, repressor, reversion, RNA, segregation, selection, sex chromosome, sex limited, syngeneic, synapsis, telophase, telosynapsis, template, transcript ion, transduction, transmutation, triploidy, trisomy, variance, X-linked, Y-linked, zygonema, zygotene
genetically different: allogeneic

genital diseases: balanitis,
balanoposthitis, eunuchoidism,
gonorrhea, hypospadias, Leber's
congenital amaurosis, leukorrhea,
pelvic inflammatory disease,
phimosis, urethritis
See also venereal diseases
genital examination: colposcopy
genitals: genito-, clitoris, cunnus,
fallopian tubes, labia major, labia
minor, muliebria, ovary, penis,
prostate, pudendum, scrotum,
testes, uterus, vulva
genitals, external, pain: pudendagra
genitals, fear of: eurotophobia
genitals, female, surgery of:
gynoplastics
genitals, small: microgenitalism
germ: blasto-, bacillus, bacterium,
microbe, microorganism, pathogen,
virus
German measles: rubella, roeteln
germ-free: axenic, sterile
germicide: antiseptic, bactericide,
disinfectant, fumigant,
microbicide
germinate: develop, grow, pullulate
germ layers: ectoderm, entoderm,
mesoderm
germs, fear of: microphobia
gestation: gravidity, incubation,
pregnancy
gestation, extrauterine: ectopic,
metacyesis
gesture, inability to: amimia
gestures, imitate: echokinesia,
echopraxia
ghosts, fear of: phasmophobia
gingiva: ulo-, ule-
girdle: cingulate, truss, zona, zone,
zoster
girdle pain: zonesthesia
girl: female
girls, fear of: parthenophobia
give birth: parturition
gland abnormality: adenectopia

gland activity, deficient: adenasthenia
gland activity, excessive:
adenohypersthenia
gland diseases: adenoma, adenopathy,
adenosis
gland enlargement: adenomegaly,
adenoncus, adenopathy,
hyperadenosis
glanders: farcy
gland growth: adenomatosis
gland hardening: adenosclerosis
gland inflammation: acinitis, adenitis,
adenocellulitis, buboadenitis,
enteradenitis, paradenitis,
periadenitis
glandlike: adeniform, adenoid,
adenose, lymphoid
gland obstruction: adenemphraxis
gland pain: adenalgia, adenodynia
gland removal: adenectomy
glands: aden-, adeni-, adeno-,
-adenia, acinous, adrenal, anterior,
apocrine, areolar, eccrine,
endocrine, exocrine, lacrimal,
meibomian, nabothian, pancreas,
parathyroid, parotid, pineal body,
pituitary (hypophysis), prostate,
pyloric, salivary, sebaceous, serous,
sudoriferous, thyroid, thymus
glands, absence: anadenia
glands, originating in: adenogenous
glands, sex, lack of: agonadism
glands, study of: adenology,
endocrinology
gland softening: adenomalacia
gland stimulator: succagogue
gland therapy: cytotherapy,
organotherapy
gland tumorlike: adenomatoid
gland tumors: acinic cell
adenoacanthoma, adenocarcinoma,
adenocele, adenochondroma,
adenocyst, adenocystoma,
adenoepithelioma, adenofibroma,
adenolipoma, adenoma,
adenomyoma, adenomyosis,
adenosarcoma,
adenosarcorhabdomyoma,
cystadenoma

glandular activity, deficient:
adenasthenia
glandular fever: infectious
mononucleosis
glass: hyal-, hyalo-
glass, fear of: crystallophobia
glass, fear of touching:
crystallophobia, hyalophobia
glass-eating: hyalophagia
glasses: bifocals, eyeglasses, lens,
ocular, spectacles, trifocals, ultex
glasslike: hyaloid
glassy: hyaline, vitreous
glaucoma: buphthalmia,
hydrophthalmos
glaucoma therapy: acetazolamide,
betaxolol, colforsin, demecarium,
dichlorphenamide, dipivefrin,
echothiophate, epinephine,
glycerin, isoflurophate, mannitol,
methazolamide, physostigmine,
pilocarpine, pirnabine, timolol,
urea
globe-shaped: globule, spheroid
globulin, excessive: hyperglobulinemia
glucocorticoids: amcinonide,
beclomethasone, betamethasone,
carbenoxolone, clocortolone,
cloprednol, corticotropin, cortisone,
cortivazol, descinolone,
dexamethasone, diflucortolone,
flucinonide, flucloronide,
flucortolone, flumethasone,
flunisolide, fluorometholone,
fluperolone, fluprednisolone,
flurandrenolide, formocortal,
hydrocortisone, medrysone,
methylprednisolone, nivazol,
paramethasone, prednicarbate,
prednisolone, prednisone,
prednival, ticarbesone, tralonide,
triamcinolone
glucose, abnormal: glucopenia,
glucosuria, hyperglycemia,
hypoglycemia
glue ear: chronic otitis media with
effusion

gluelike: glio-
gluey: adhesive, albuminous, mucous,
viscid
gluten allergy: celiac disease
gluttony: acoria, polyphagia
glycogen storage diseases:
amylopectinosis, Andersen's
disease, Cori's disease, dextrinosis,
glycogenosis, McArdle's disease,
Pompe's disease, von Gierke's
disease
See also metabolism diseases
God, fear of: theophobia
goggle-eyed: exophthalmic
goiter: exophthalmic, Graves' disease
goiter causing: goitrogen
goiter inflammation: peristrumitis,
perithyroiditis
gold deposition: chrysiasis
gold therapy: aurotherapy,
chrysotherapy, oleochrysotherapy
gonadal diseases: amenorrhea,
cryptorchidism, dysgenesis,
eunuchoidism, hypergonadism,
hypogonadism, Kallmann
syndrome, Klinefelter syndrome,
pseudoprecocity, Turner syndrome
gonads: ovary, testis
gonads, absence: agonadism
gonococci, in blood: gonococcemia,
gonohemia
good: eu-
goose bumps: horri-, arrector pili,
cutis anserina, formication,
pilation, piloerection, pilomotor
reflex
gout: podagra
gout, nonjoint: abarticular
gout, of hand: cheiraga
gout, of elbow: anconagra
gout therapy: allopurinol, antarthritic,
arthrifuge, colchicine, fenoprofen,
ibuprofen, indomethacin,
naproxen, oxyphenbutazone,
phenbutazone, piroxicam,
probenicid, sulfinpyrazone, sulindac

graft: allograft, allotransplantation, autograft, autotransplantation, dermatoheteroplasty, heteroautoplasty, heterograft, hetero-osteoplasty, heteroplasty, homeo-osteoplasty, homograft, implant, isograft, syngenesioplasty, transplant, xenograft, zoografting, zooplasty

grain itch: acarodermatitis

grain-shaped: sesamoid

granulation tissue: acestoma

granules: Nissl bodies

granules, condition of: granulocytopenia, granuloma, granulopenia, granulopoiesis, granulosis

granuloma diseases: granulomatosis, sarcoidosis

grapelike: racemose

grape-shaped: aciniform, botryoid, staphyline

grape therapy: ampelotherapy

grasping: awareness, perception, prehension

grass: cannabis, hashish, marijuana

grating: crepitation

gravel-like: arenaceous, arenoid

gravity, fear of: barophobia

gray: canescent, cineritious, pallid

gray hair: achromotrichia, canities, hemicanities, poliosis

gray matter: polio-, cinerea

gray matter disease: poliodystrophy, polioencephalopathy, poliomyelopathy

gray matter destruction: polioclastic

gray matter inflammation: polioencephalitis, polioencephalomeningomyelitis, polioencephalomyelitis, poliomyelitis, poliomyeloencephalitis

great: mega-, megalo-, -megaly, vastus

great toe: hallux

greedy: pleonexia

green: chlor-

green blindness: achloropsia, aglaukopsia, chloropsia, daltonism, deuteranopia, protanopia, xanthocyanopsia

green cancer: chloroma

grin: risus

grin, abnormal: risus sardonicus

grind: mortar and pestle, pulverize

grind, of teeth: bruxism, bruxomania, brychomania, odontoprisis

grinder: molar tooth

gripes: colic-

grippe: influenza

gristle: cartilage

gritty: acervulus, arenaceous, granular, psammous, pulverous, sabulous, sandy, tophaceous

grocer's itch: hand eczema

groggy: stupor

groin: inguen

groove: canal, channel, cleft, crevice, fissure, furrow, sulcus, vallecula

grooves, three: trisulcate

grotesque: aberrant, abnormal, anomalous, deviant, malformed, monster

ground itch: ancylostomiasis

group: agglutination, aggregation, classification, clumping, cluster, genus, species, subdivision, variety

group, development of: phylogeny

growth: auxo-, polyp-, -trophy, accretion, anabolism, anachronobiology, auxesis, cyst, enlargement, germination, intumescence, maturation, tumescence, tumor

growth, abnormal: cacogenesis, cancer, chondrodysplasia, chondrodystrophy, dyschondroplasia, enchondromatosis, malignancy, Ollier's disease, polyp, tumor

growth, new: neoplasm

growth, rapid: proliferation
growth, science of: auxanology
growth, secondary: metatasis
growth, slow: indolent
growth, toward sun: heliotropism
growth, without oxygen: anaerobic
growth retardation: hypogenesis,
    nanism
grow together: accretion, adhesion,
    coalesce
grow worse: decay, degenerate,
    deteriorate, malignant, weaken
guide: mandrin, prototype
gullet: esophagus
gum: euo-, ule-, gingiva
gum arabic: acacia
gum bleeding: oulorrhagia,
    ulemorrhagia, ulorrhagia, ulorrhea
gumboil: gingival abscess, parulis
gum disease: gingivitis, ulocace
gum incision: ulotomy
gum inflammation: gingivitis,
    peridentitis, ulitis, uloglossitis
gum irritation: ulaganactesis
gum massage: ulotripsis
gum pain: gingivalgia, ulalgia
gum shrinkage: recession, ulatrophy
gum surgery: ulectomy
gum tissue removal: gingivectomy,
    ulectomy
gum tumor: ulocarcinoma, uloncus
gush: effusion, hemorrhage
gut: abdomen, belly, intestines

H

habit: addiction, dependence, mania
habit, bad: cacoethes
habit spasm: tic
Hageman factor: Factor XII
hair: pilo-, trichi-, tricho-, capillus,
    crinis, pile, pilus, pubes, tragi
hair, axillary: hirci
hair, brittle: sclerothrix, sclerotrichia,
    trichatrophia, trichorrhexis,
    tricoclasia

hair, excessive: Achard-Thiers
    syndrome, hirsutism,
    hypertrichosis, pilosis, polytrichosis,
    trichauxis
hair, fear of: hypertrichophobia,
    trichopathophobia, trichophobia
hair, habit of breaking off:
    trichokryptomania,
    trichorrhexomania
hair, ingrown: pilus incarnatus
hair, lack of: alopecia, atrichosis,
    baldness, oligotrichia, ophiasis
hair, matted: plica polonica,
    trichomatosis
hair, pull out: trichologia,
    trichotillomania
hair, soft: lanugo, pubescence
hair, stiff: seta, vibrissae
hair, straight: leiotrichous, lissotrichy
hair, study of: trichology
hair, white: canities, leukotrichia,
    poliosis
hairball: bezoar, pilobezoar,
    trichobezoar, trichophytobezoar
hair cycle: anagen, catagen, telogen
hair diseases: districhiasis,
    hypotrichosis, Menkes kinky hair
    syndrome, monilethrix,
    paratrichosis, sclerotrichia,
    trichomycosis, trichonosis,
    trichopathy, trichosis,
    trichosporosis
hair eating: trichophagia
hair examination: trichoscopy
hair follicle inflammation:
    epifolliculitis, folliculitis,
    perifolliculitis, Quinquaud's disease,
    sycosis
hair follicle disease: trichocryptosis
hair formation: piliation
hair growth stimulant: trichogenous,
    trychophytic
hairlike: celia, cercus, piliform,
    trichoid
hair loss: defluvium capillorum,
    trichomodesis, trichorrhea

hair nutrition: trichotrophy
hair on fetus: lanugo
hair removal: decalvant, depilation, electrolysis, epilation, epipilatory
hair splitting: clastothrix, distrix, schizotrichia, scissura pilorum, trichorrhexis
hairy: hirsutism, pileous, pilose, pilous
hairy tongue: glossophytia, trichoglossia
half: demi-, hemi-, semi-
half-breed: crossbreeding, hybrid
half-moon: lunula
half-wit: idiot, imbecile, mental retardation, moron
hallucination: aberration, acousma, deja vu, delusion, disorientation, fantasy, illusion, oneirism, pseudoblepsis, pseudopsia, psychodelic, psychosensory, psychotomimetic
halo: areola, corona
hammer: malleus, plessor
hamstrings: biceps femoris, semimembranosus, semitendenosus
hand: cheir-, cheiro-, chir-, chiro-, carpus, extremity, main, manus, metacarpus, phalanges
    See also digit
hand, abnormal: atelocheiria, bidactyly, malleation, polyphalangism
hand, back of: opisthenar
hand, between thumb and index finger: anatomical snuffbox, tabatiere anatomique
hand, excessive sweating: acrohyperhidrosis
hand, large: cheiromegaly, macrocheiria
hand, small: microcheiria
handful: pugil
handicap: disability, impairment
hand lines: palmar creases, simian creases
hand pain: cheiralgia, chiralgia

hand plastic surgery: cheiroplasty
hands, absence of: acheiria, acheiropody, achiria
hands, equal use of: ambidexterity, bimanual
hands, poor use of: ambilevosity
hands and feet, abnormality: athetosis, mobile spasm, posthemiplegic chorea
hand spasm: cheirospasm, chirismus, chirospasm
hand tremor: asterixis
hanging: pendulous
hangnail: agnail
hangover: crapulence
hard: sclero-, adamantine, turgid
hardening: calcification, coagulation, induration, ossify, sclerosis
hardening, abnormal: calcinosis
hardening of arteries: atherosclerous, arteriosclerosis
hare eye: lagophthalmos
harelip: cleft lip
harlequin fetus: ichthyosis congenita
harmful: corrosive, lethal, noxious, pernicious, poisonous, septic, toxic, virulent
harmless: benign, innocuous, innoxious
haunch: buttocks, hips, iliac
hay fever: pollinosis, rhinitis
head: capit-, cephal-, -cephalia, cephalo-, caput, cephalic, cranium, face, sinciput, skull, temple
head, abnormal: atelocephalous, ateloencephalia, cephalodactyly, cephalomelus, cephalonia, cephalothoracopagus, perocephalus, scaphocephaly
head, away from: cephalocaudad
head, back of: occipital, occiput
head, clearing: cephalocathartic
head, fetal and maternal pelvis: cephalopelvic
head, front of: face, frons, metropic, procephalic
head, large: cephalonia, macrocephaly, megalocephaly

head, narrow: sternocephaly
hear, removal: decapitation,
    decollation, detruncation
head, round: trochocephalia
head, short: brachycephaly,
    hyperbrachycephaly
head, small: leptocephaly,
    microcephaly, nanocephalism
head, top of: corona capitis, crown,
    vertex
head, toward: cephalad, craniad
head, watery accumulation:
    cephalhydrocele
headache: caphalagra, cephalalgia,
    cephalea, cephalodynia, clavus,
    cluster, encephalalgia, hemicrania,
    migraine
head and chest: cephalothoracic
head blow: concussion
head development: cephalization,
    cephalogenesis
head disease: cephalopathy
head edema: cephaledema,
    hydrocephalus
head examination: cephalography,
    cephaloscopy
head hemorrhage: cephalhematoma,
    cephalohematoma
headless: acephalo-, abrachiocephalia,
    acephalobrachia, acephalus,
    acephaly, hemicephalus
head lice: pediculosis capitis
head measurement: cephalic index,
    cephalometry
head measurement, instrument:
    cephalometer
head movement: cephalogyric,
    cephalomotor, gyrospasm
head muscles: semispinalis,
    sternocleiromastoid, temporal
head muscles, paralysis: cephaloplegia
head protrusion: cephalocele, inion
head puncture: cephalocentesis
heads, two: ancipital, dicephalism
head-shaped: capitate
head to tail: cephalocaudal

head tumor: cephalhematocele,
    cephalohematocele
heal: cure, palliate, regenerate,
    rehabilitate, repair, resuscitate,
    therapy, treatment
healing: cicatrization, curative, first
    intention, medicinal, recuperating,
    sanative, second intention,
    therapeutic,.third intention
healing, normally: euplastic
health, excessive concern for:
    hygieiolatry, hypochondria
health, good: euphoria
health, study of: hygieiology, hygiene
healthful: hygienic, salubrious,
    salutary, sanitary
health restoration: analepsis
heaped: aggregated, clot, clump,
    cluster, concentration,
    conglomerate
hearing: acou-, -acousia, acu-, -acusia,
    audio-, acousia, acoustics, audition,
    auditory, ausculatation
    See also ear
hearing, acute: hyperacusis
hearing, normal: acusis
hearing, painful: odynacusis
hearing, science of: audiology
hearing, sense of: acouesthesia
hearing diseases: pseudacousma,
    pseudacusis, psychic deafness,
    paracusis
hearing dullness: bradyacusia
hearing impairment: amblyacousia,
    anacousia, anacroasia, bradyecoia,
    conductive loss, deafness,
    dysacousia, paracusis, presbyacusis,
    sensorineural
hearing specialist: audiologist
hearing test: audiometry, Bekesy's,
    evoked potential, Rinne,
    Schwabach, Weber
heart: card-, cardia-, cardio-, cardiac,
    cor, epicardium, myocardium,
    endocardium
heart, abnormal: atelocardia

heart, absent: acardia
heart, air in: pneumatocardia
heart, athlete's: enlarged heart
heart, electric shock to: defibrillation
heart, enlarged: cardiectasis,
    cardiohepatomegaly, cardiomegaly,
    cor pulmonale, megacardia,
    megalocardia
heart, origin in: cardiogenic
heart, right: dextrocardia
heart, small: microcardia
heart, study of: cardiology
heart area: antecardium, precardium
heart atrophy: acardiotrophia
heart attack: cardiovascular disease,
    myocardial infarction
heartbeat, abnormal: allorhythmia,
    anisorhythmia, arrhythmia, atrial
    fibrillation, polycrotism, sick sinus
    syndrome
heartbeat, rapid: gallop rhythm,
    neurocirculatory asthenia,
    palpitations, tachycardia,
    tachyrhythmia
heartbeat, rhythmic: pulsatile,
    pulsation, pulse, throbbing
heartbeat, slow: brachycardia,
    bradycardia, bradyrhythmia,
    oligocardia
heartburn: brash, cardialgia,
    dyspepsia, gastric distress,
    gastroesophageal reflux,
    indigestion, peratodynia, pyrosis
heart calculus: cardiolith
heart chambers: atrium, ventricle
heart constriction: cardiostenosis
heart contraction: fibrillation, systole
heart contraction, absent: asystole
heart degeneration: cardiomyoliposis,
    cardionecrosis
heart disease, fear of: cardiophobia
heart disease classification: Killip, New
    York Heart Association
heart diseases: aneurysm, angina
    pectoris, aortic regurgitation,
    aortic valve stenosis, arrhythmias,
    atrial fibrillation, atrial flutter,
    atrial septal defect,
    atrioventricular block, bifascicular

block, bundle branch block, cardiac
arrest, cardiomyopathy,
cardioneurosis, cardiopathy,
coarctation of the aorta, congestive
heart failure, cor biloculare, cor
pulmonale, cor triatriatum, cor
triloculare biatriatum, Ebstein's
anomaly, Eisenmenger's syndrome,
endocarditis, hemiblock,
hemipericardium, Lutembacher's
syndrome, mitral regurgitation,
mitral stenosis, myocardial
infarction, myocardiosis,
myocardosis, myocele, patent
ductus arteriosus, patent foramen
ovale, pericardial tamponade,
pneumohemopericardium,
pneumohydropericardium,
pneumopericardium,
pneumopyopericardium,
polyarteritis nodosa, presbycardia,
pulmonic stenosis, rheumatic,
tetralogy of Fallot, truncus
arteriosus, valvular heart disease,
ventricular septal defect, Wolff-
Parkinson-White syndrome
    See also congenital diseases
heart displacement: bathycardia,
    cardioptosis, ectocardia,
    trochocardia
heart enlargement: bucardia,
    cardiectasia, cardiomegaly,
    megacardia
heart examination: angiocardiography,
    angiography, apexcardiography,
    ballistocardiography, cardiography,
    cardioscopy, catheterization,
    Doppler cardiography,
    echocardiography,
    electrocardiography, Holter
    monitoring, phonocardiography,
    stress test
heart failure: asystole, cardiac arrest
heart hardening: cardiosclerosis
heart hernia: cardiocele
heart incision: cardiotomy

heart inflammation: angiocarditis, cardiopericarditis, cardiovalvulitis, carditis, endocarditis, endomyocarditis, endopericarditis, endoperimyocarditis, ethmocarditis, myocarditis, myoendocarditis, myopericarditis, pancarditis, pericarditis, perimyoendocarditis, pneumopericarditis, pyopericarditis, pyopneumopericarditis, thromboendocarditis

heartlike: cardioid

heart-lung machine: extracorporeal circulation

heart membranes: pericardium, epicardium, endocardium

heart muscle: myocardium

heart muscle disease: cardiomyopathy

heart pain: angina, cardialgia, cardiodynia

heart paralysis: cardioplegia

heart pill: digitalis

heart poisoning: cardiotoxic

heart puncture: cardiocentesis, cardiopuncture, pericardiocentesis

heart rate: *See* heartbeat

heart relaxation: diastole

heart rhythm restored: cardioversion

heart rupture: cardiorrhexis

heart-shaped: cordate, cordiform

heart softening: cardiomalacia

heart specialist: cardiologist

heart stimulants: dobutamine, dopamine, epinephrine, isoproterenol

heart surgery: angioplasty, Beck operation, Blalock-Taussig procedure, bypass, cardiolysis, cardioplasty, commissurotomy, coronary bypass, endarterectomy, Mustard, open-heart, percutaneous transluminal coronary angioplasty, shunting, transplantation, valve replacement

heart suturing: cardiomyopexy, cardiorrhaphy

heart therapy: acebutolol, actodigin, amrinone, atenolol, butopamine, captopril, carbazeran, cardiotherapy, cardiotonic, deslanoside, digitalis, digitoxin, digoxin, enoximone, hydralazine, isomazole, isosorbide, metoprolol, milrinone, nadolol, nitroglycerin, nitroprusside, oxprenolol, pelrinone, phentolamine, piroximone, prazosin, propranolol, proscillaridin, quazinone, sulfinpyrazone, tazolol, timolol

heart tumors: myxoma, rhabdomyoma

heart valves: aortic, bicuspid, mitral, semilunar, tricuspid

heart weakness: amyocardia, myasthenia cordis

heat: pyro-, therm-, thermo-, calefacient, calor, calorie, estruation, estrus, fever, flush, pyrexia

heat, fear of: thermophobia

heat conditions: exhaustion, heatstroke, hyperpyremia, hyperthermia, siriasis, stroke, sunstroke

heat insensitive: thermanalgesia, thermanesthesia, thermoresistant, thermostabile

heat loss: hypothermia, thermolysis, thermosteresia

heat measurement: calorimetry, thermography, thermometry

heat pain: thermalgesia, thermohyperalgesia

heat poison: thermotoxin

heat production: calorific, thermogenesis

heat production, stopped: thermoinhibitory

heat regulating: thermotaxic

heat sensitive: thermolabile

heat sensitivity: hyperthermalgesia, hyperthermoesthesia, thermalgesia, thermesthesia, thermoesthesia

heat sensitivity disorders:
ardanesthesia, caumesthesia,
hyperthermalgesia,
thermanalgesia, thermanesthesia,
thermhyperesthesia,
thermoanalgesia,
thermoanesthesia,
thermohyperesthesia,
thermohypesthesia
heatstroke: hyperpyrexia, insolation,
siriasis, thermoplegia
heat therapy: chauffage, diathermy,
fomentation, galvanothermy,
hyperpyrexia, hyperthermia,
ignipuncture, poultice, pyronyxis,
pyropuncture, radiothermy,
thermocauterectomy,
thermocautery, thermocoagulation,
thermopenetration,
thermoradiotherapy,
thermotherapy, transthermia
heat treatment, study of:
thermatology
heave: disgorge, regurgitate, retch,
vomit
heavy: bary-, obese
heavy physique: endomorph
heel: calcaneous, calcar pedis, calx
heel pain: calcaneodynia, calcanodynia,
talalgia
height: hypso-
heights, fear of: acrophobia,
batophobia, hypsophobia
helmet-shaped: galea
hemoglobin, lack of: hypochromia,
oligochromemia
hemoglobin in urine: hemoglobinuria
hemoglobin release: hemolysis
hemophilia A: Factor VIII deficiency
hemophilia B: Factor IX deficiency
hemophilia C: Factor XI deficiency
hemorrhage: -rrhage, hematocele,
hematorrhea
See also bleeding
hemorrhage, stopping: astringent,
hemostat, staunch, styptic

hemorrhage in abdomen:
hematoperitoneum
hemorrhage in brain:
hematencephalon
hemorrhage in cyst: hematocyst
hemorrhage in spinal cord:
hematomelia, hematorrhachis
hemorrhage in umbilical hernia:
hematomphalocele
hemorrhage in uterus: hematometra
hemorrhoid removal:
hemorrhoidectomy
hemostatic: aminocaproic acid,
ethamsylate, oxamarin, sulmarin,
thrombin, tranexamic acid
henbane: hyoscyamus
hereditary: congenital, genetic,
inborn, inherited, innate,
transmissible
See also genetics
hereditary diseases: acatalasia,
alkaptonuria, amaurotic familial
idiocy, amyloidosis, aniridia,
anophthalmos, antitrypsin
deficiency, argenosuccinic aciduria,
arthrodysplasia,
aspartylglycosaminuria, Bloom's
syndrome, cardiomyopathy,
cerebroretinal angiomatosis,
Charcot-Marie-Tooth atrophy,
Chediak-Higashi syndrome,
chondrodystrophia calcificans
congenita, cleidocranial dysostosis,
coloboma, coproporphyria,
cretinism, craniorachischisis,
craniosynostosis, cri du chat
syndrome, Crigler-Najjar
syndrome, cutis verticis gyrata,
cystathioninuria, cystic fibrosis,
diabetes insipidus, distichiasis,
Dubin-Johnson syndrome,
Dubowitz syndrome, Duchenne
muscular dystrophy, dysautonomia,
dyschondrosteosis, Ellis-van
Creveld syndrome, Fabry disease,
familial polyposis, Fanconi's
anemia, Friedreich's ataxia,
fucosidosis, galactosemia, Gaucher's

disease, Gilbert's syndrome,
glycogen storage disease, Hartnup
disease, histidinemia, Huntington's
chorea, hypofibrinogenemia,
hypophosphatasia, keratoconus,
Klinefelter's syndrome, Laurence-
Moon-Biedl syndrome, Lesch-
Nyhan syndrome, Marfan's
syndrome, Marshall syndrome,
melorheostosis, Menkes kinky hair
syndrome, methemoglobulinemia,
Mondini malformation,
mucopolysaccharidosis, Naegel's
syndrome, Netherton's syndrome,
Nezelof's syndrome, Niemann-Pick
disease, Noonan's syndrome,
Pendred's syndrome, Peutz-
Jeghers syndrome, Pfeiffer's
syndrome, phenylketonuria,
proteinosis, Rendu-Osler-Weber
syndrome, sickle cell thalassemia,
Sipple's syndrome, Stumpell's
disease, Tay-Sachs disease, Turner's
syndrome, Verner-Morrison islet
cell tumor syndrome, von Hippel-
Lindau disease, xanthinuria,
xanthomatosis
heredity: genes, genetic makeup,
genetics, inheritance
heritage: pedigree, strain
hermaphroditism: amphigonadism,
androgyne, bisexual, gynander,
intersexual,
pseudohermaphroditism,
transsexual
hernia: bubonocele, diaphragmatic,
entocele, epiplocele,
epiplomphalocele,
epiplosarcomphalocele,
epiploscheocele, exomphalos,
inguinal, rupture
hernia, study of: herniology
hernia, of scrotum: orchiocele,
orchioscheocele
hernia device: truss
hernia reduction: taxis

hernia surgery: Bassini's operation,
celology, hernioplasty, herniotomy,
kelotomy
hernia suturing: herniorrhaphy
herpeslike: herpetiform
hiatus: synapse
hiccup: singultus, spasmalygmus
hidden: crypt-, crypto-, cryptic,
latent, occult
hidebound disease: scleroderma
high blood pressure: hyperpiesia,
hypertension
high blood pressure treatment:
antihypertensive
high places, fear of: acrophobia
high point: acme, fastigium
high-strung: hyperactive, neurotic
high temperature: hyperthermia,
pyrexia
hinge joint: ginglymus, synovial
hip: coxa, innominate bone, ilium,
ischium, pubis
hip joint disease: coxarthropathy
hip joint inflammation: coxarthria,
coxarthritis, coxitis
hip pain: coxalgia, coxodynia,
ischialgia, ischioneuralgia, sciatica
hip replacement: arthroplasty,
hemiarthroplasty
hiss: sibilant, sibilismus
histamine suppressor: antihistamine
hives: uredo, urticaria
hoarseness: dysphonia, gutteral
hobnail liver: cirrhosis
hole: cavity, cleft, fenestra, fissure,
foramen, fossa, hiatus, orifice,
perforation, pore, puncture, sinus,
sulcus
hollow: cav-, alveolus, caverna, cavity,
depression, excavation, hof,
incisure, lacuna, socket
hollowback: lordosis
hollow organ, base of: fundus
hollow spaces: cavernous, cavity
home, fear of: oikophobia
home, leaving: apodemialgia

homesickness: nostalgia
homogenous: hol-, holo-
honey: mel-
honeycombed: alveolate, faveolate
hook-shaped: ancistroid, ancyroid,
    arc, curvature, flexura, hamular,
    unciform, uncinate, uncus
hookworm: Ancylostoma, Necator,
    Uncinaria
hookworm disease: ancylostomiasis,
    necatoriasis, uncinariasis
horizontal: abscissa, prone
hormone production: hormogenic,
    hormopoiesis, hormotropic
hormone suppressant: anahormone
hormones: adrenocorticotrophic,
    aldosterone, andrin, androgen,
    androsterone, antidiuretic,
    calcitonin, cholecystokinin,
    corticosterone, cortisol, cortisone,
    dehydroepiandrosterone,
    epinephrine, estradiol, estriol,
    estrogen, estrone, follicle-
    stimulating, gastrin, growth,
    hydrocortisone, insulin, luteinizing,
    melatonin, norepinephrine,
    oxytocin, parathormone,
    parathyroxin, progesterone,
    progestin, prolactin, relaxin,
    secretin, serotonin, somatotrophin,
    testosterone, thymosin, thyroid-
    stimulating, thyrotropin,
    thyroxine, vasopressin
hormones, study of: hormonology
hormone therapy: endocrinotherapy
horn: callus, corn, cornu
horny: kerat-, kerato-, corneous,
    indurated, keratose, ossified
horny growth: callosity, callus,
    keratoderma, keratoma,
    keratonosis, keratosis
horny skin layer: stratum corneum
horny skin layer, dissolution:
    keratolysis
horny tissue: cerato-, kerato-
horny tissue development:
    keratinization, keratogenesis,
    keratogenous

horseshoe-shaped: hyoid
hospital: asylum, clinic, convalescent
    home, dispensary, halfway house,
    hospice, infirmary, medical center,
    nursing care facility, nursing
    home, polyclinic, sanatorium,
    sanitarium
hospital-acquired: nosocomial
hostile behavior: aggression
hot: calenture, pyretic, radioactive
Hottentot bustle: steatopygia
house, fear of: domatophobia
housemaid's knee: prepatellar bursitis
hovering sensation: anakatesthesia
huge: giga-, gigantism
humans, fear of: anthropophobia
humerus projection: epitrochlea
humming noise: bourdonnement
hump: gibbus, lump, node,
    protuberance
humpback: gibbous, kyphosis, scoliosis
hunger: limo-, acoria, appetite,
    bulimia, cynorexia,
    gastralgokenosis, hyperorexia,
    limosis, lycorexia, polyphagia
    See also appetite, eating disorders,
    food
hunger cure: nestotherapy
hurt: See pain
hyaline in urine: hyalinuria
hyaline membrane disease: respiratory
    distress syndrome
hybrid: alloy, compound,
    conglomerate, crossbreeding
hydrocarbon: -ane
hydrocarbons, open-chained: aliphatic
hydrochloric acid, decreased:
    hypochlorhydria
hydrochloric acid, excess:
    hyperchlorhydria
hydrogen ion, increased in blood:
    acidemia, acidosis
hydrophobia: rabies
hygiene: disinfection, douch, oral
    hygiene, preventive medicine,
    public health, sanitation, sterilize

hymen, imperforate: hematocolpos, hematometra, mucocolpos
hymen rupture: defloration
hypersensitivity reaction: anaphylactic shock, type I hypersensitivity, cell-mediated hypersensitivity, cytotoxic hypersensitivity, immune complex hypersensitivity
hypersensitivity treatment: antihistamine
hypertension: *See* high blood pressure
hypertension, idiopathic: essential hypertension
hypnosis: catalepsy, coma, somnolence, sopor, unconsciousness
hypnotics: allobarbital, alonimid, amobarbital, brotizolam, butabarbital, capuride, carbocloral, chloral hydrate, clorethate, etomidate, flunitrazepam, flurazepam, fosazepam, lormetazepam, mecloqualone, methaqualone, nisobamate, nitrazepam, paraldehyde, pentobarbital, perlapine, phenobarbital, quazepam, roletamide, secobarbital, thalidomide, triazolam, triclofos
hypnotic suggestion: teleotherapeutics
hypnotism: autosuggestion, mesmerism
hypobranchial eminence: furcula
hypochondria: depressed, hypochondriasis, melancholia, psychoneurotic
hypotensives: dicirenone, viprostol
hysterectomy, subtotal: myohysterectomy
hysteria: convulsion, dancing mania, paroxysm, pseudochorea, seizure, spasm
hysteria preventive: anthysteric, antihysteric

I

ice, eating: pagophagia
ideas, fear of: ideaphobia
identical: iso-
identical twins: monozygotic twins
identity confusion: dissociative disorder
idiocy: feeblemindedness, mental deficiency, mental retardation
idiot: ament, feebleminded, mentally deficient, mentally retarded
ileum: ileo-, ileac, Meckel's diverticulum
ileum excision: ileectomy
ileum incision: ileocolotomy, ileotomy
ileum inflammation: Crohn's disease, ileitis, ileocolitis
ileum surgery: ileocecostomy, ileocolostomy, ileoileostomy, ileoproctostomy, ileorectostomy, ileosigmoidostomy, ileostomy, ileosystostomy, ileotransversostomy
ileum suturing: ileorrhapy
iliac gland abscess: poradenitis
ilium: ilio-
ill: cac-, caci-, caco-, mal-, disease, indisposed, infirm, invalid
ill-being: cenesthopathia
ill health: cachexia
illness: noso-, patho-, affliction, disability, disease, disorder, infection, malady, mental disorder, neurosis, psychosis
illness, caused by doctors: iatrogenic, odontiatrogenic
illness, caused in hospital: nosocomial
illness, fear of: nosophobia
ill-smelling: miasmic, putrid, rancid
illuminate: irradiate, phosphorescent
illusion: delusion, fantasy, hallucination, phantasm
image: spectro-, imago
imbecilic: anile, mentally deficient, mentally retarded

imitation: clone, echokinesia, echolalia, echomimia, echomotism, echopathy, echophrasia, echopraxia, malingering, mimesis, mimicry, simulation

immature: blasto-, blast, abortive, embryonic, juvenile, rudimentary

immediately: stat

immune response stimulator: adjuvant

immunity: inoculation, insusceptibility, premunition, vaccinate

immunity, decreasing: anaphylactic, anti-immune

immunity, inducing: immunogenic

immunity, study of: immunology, immunopathology

immunodeficiency: anergy

immunoglobulins: A, D, E, G, M; antibody

immunosuppressants: azathioprine, betamethasone, chlorambucil, corticotropin, cortisone, cyclophosphamide, cyclosporine, dexamethasone, fanetizole, frentizole, hydrocortisone, mercaptopurine, methylprednisolone, paramethasone, prednisolone, prednisone, ristianol, thymopentin, triamcinolone

impaired: deficient, disabled, mentally retarded

impaired smell: dysosmia

impaired thinking: dyslogia

impairment: disability, vitiation

imperceptible: microscopic

imperfect: atelo-, defect

imperforate: atreto-

imperforate anus: proctatresia

imperforate hymen: hematocolpos, hematometra, mucocolpos

impetigo: Ritter's disease

impetus: impulse

implantation: impregnation, nidation

impotence: agenesis, infecundity, infertility, sterility

impregnation: conception, fecundation, fertilize, insemination, procreation, saturation, syllepsis

improve: convalesce, heal, recuperate

impulse, passage of: acetylcholine, neurotransmitter

impure: contaminated, feculent, infected, turbid

impurities, removal: cleanse, depurant, purify

in: em-, en-, in-

inactive: anergic, dormant, inanimate, indolent, inert, latent, lifeless, placebo, quiescent, torpid, undeveloped

in addition to: extra-

inborn: congenital, hereditary, inbred, inherent, innate, intrinsic

incapacity: disability, handicap, mental retardation

incision: -tomy, celiotomy, gastronomy, kerf, laparotomy
    See also individual organs

incomplete: atelo-

incontinence: -cratia, encopresis, enuresis, gatism, scoracratia, uracratia

incoordinated: ataxia, dyssynergia

increase: auxo-, distend, elevate, generate, germinate, pullulate, reproduce, swell
    See also growth

incurable: terminal

indecisive: folie du doute

indentation: cavity, cleft, recess

index case: proband, propositus

India rubber man: Ehlers-Danlos syndrome

indication: sign, symptom

indigestion: cacochylia, cardialgia, dyspepsia, gastric distress, hyperpepsia, nausea, pyrosis

indigestion, acid: hyperchlorhydria

indisposed: bedridded, disabled, hospitalized, ill

individual: idio-
    See also self

individual, development of: ontogeny
induced abortion: abactio
induration: sclerosis
inebriate: alcoholic, crapulent, intoxicated
inert: comatose, inactive, inanimate, nonviable, supine, somnolent, torpid, unconscious
infant: brepho-, neonate, newborn
infant cry, first: vagitus
infantile paralysis: poliomyelitis
infection: contagion, contamination, bacillus, disease, microbism, multiinfection, polyinfection, virus
infection, ameba: amebiasis
infection, fear of: molysmophobia
infection, protection against: alexeteric, inoculation, vaccination
infection outbreak: epidemic, pandemic, plague
infection preventive: antisepsis, antiserum, inoculation, vaccine
infection product: pus
infectious: communicable, contagious, plague, superinfection, transmissible, virulent
infectious agent: contagium, dengue
infectious diseases: anthrax, Argentine hemorrhagic fever, aspergillosis, bacteremia, blastomycosis, Bolivian hemorrhagic fever, Bornholm, boutonneuse fever, brucellosis, candidiasis, chickenpox, cholera, coccidioidomycosis, croup, cryptococcosis, dengue, diphtheria, dysentery, encephalitis, endocarditis, enteric fever, epidemic pleurodynia, gangrene, histoplasmosis, infectious mononucleosis, influenza, kala-azar, listeriosis, measles, meningitis, mucormycosis, mumps, otitis media, pertussis, plague, pneumonia, pox, rubella, rubeola, salmonellosis, scarlet fever, smallpox, sporotrichosis, tuberculosis, tularemia, typhoid

fever, typhus, vaccinia, Vincent's angina, viral, yellow fever
See also communicable diseases
infertile: sterile
infinity, fear of: apeirophobia
infirmary: clinic, dispensory, hospice, hospital, pharmacy, nursing home, sanatorium
infirmity: defect, disease, disorder, infection, impairment
inflamed: fester
inflammation: -itis, phlogo-, erysipelas, exanthema, hyperemia, phlegmasia, phlogosis, supporation
inflammation, glandular: adenitis
inflammation producing: phlogogenic
inflammation product: pus
inflammation symptoms: calor, dolor, rubor, tumor
inflammatory bowel disease: Crohn's disease
inflammatory therapy: anti-inflammatory, antiphlogistic
inflate: dilate, distend, swell
inflated: turgid, ventricose
influence: -trope, -tropic, -tropy
infolding: indigitation, intussusception, invagination, inversion, retroflexion
in front of: ante-, antero-, fore-, pre-, pro-
infusion: injection, inoculation, transfusion
inguinal gland inflammation: buboadenitis
inhale: aspirate, breathe in, inspire, respire
inheritance: heredity, Mendelism, pedigree
See also genetics
inheritance, female line: hologynic
inheritance, male line: holandric
inheritance, study of: genetics
inherited: congenital, familial, genetic, hereditary, trait
inherited diseases: *See* hereditary diseases

inherited tendency: instinct
inhibition: repression
injection: -clysis, inoculation,
    vaccination, vaccine
injury: noci-, traumato-, abrasion,
    bruise, contusion, laceration, lesion,
    trauma, vitiation, wound
injury, fear of: traumatophobia
inlay: facing
innate: congenital, hereditary, inborn,
    inbred, indigenous, inherited,
    organic
innermost: core, intima, marrow,
    nucleus
inner self: anima persona
innominate bone: ilium, ischium, pubis
innovation, fear of: neophobia
inoculation: immunization, vaccination
inquiry: analysis, assay, autopsy,
    examination, research, study
insanity: abalienation, dementia,
    mental illness, neurosis,
    psychoneurosis, psychosis
insanity, fear of: lyssophobia,
    maniaphobia
insects, fear of: acarophobia,
    entomophobia
insects, study of: entomology
inside: end-, endo-, ento-, intra-,
    entad, ental
insides: internal organs, viscera
    See also abdomen, intestine
inspire: breathe in, eupnea, inhale,
    respire
instep: metatarsus
instinctive: congenital, inborn, inbred,
    innate, hereditary
instruments: accelerometer,
    actinometer, adipometer,
    aeroplethysmograph, albumoscope,
    algesichronometer, algesimeter,
    algometer, altimeter, analyzers,
    anemometer, audiometer,
    autoclave, balances, blenders,
    bougie, calorimeter,
    cardiotachometer, centrifuge,
    collimator, colorimeter, colposcope,
    defibrillator, densitometer,
    desiccator, detectors, dialyzer,
dosimeter, electrocardiograph,
electroencephalograph, electrolizer,
electrometer, electromyograph,
electron microscope, endoscopes,
evaporator, fibrillator, flow meter,
galvonometer, gas analyzer,
goniometer, hemocytometer,
hydrometer, hygrometer,
hyperbaric chamber, laser,
manometer, mass spectrometer,
microscopes, microtome,
nephelometer, nuclear magnetic
imager, oscilloscope, osmometer,
pH meter, plethysmograph,
pneumotactograph, polarimeter,
radiometer, ratemeter,
refractometer, respirator,
respirometer, resuscitator,
rheometer, scales, scanners, sound,
spectrofluorometer, spectrograph,
spectrometer, spectrophotometer,
sphygomomanometer, spirometer,
stethoscope, stroboscope,
synthesizer, tachistoscope,
tachometer, thermometer,
transducer, ultrasound, vibrator,
viscometer, voltmeter
    See also surgical instruments
insufficient: oligo-
insulin, excess: hyperinsulinemia,
    hyperinsulinism, insulinemia
insulin, insufficient: diabetes mellitus,
    hypoinsulinemia
insulin overdose: glucatonia, insulin
    shock
intellectual perception: noumenon
intemperance: alcoholism, crapulence,
    dipsomania
intensifying screen: fluorescent screen
interbrain: diencephalon,
    thalamencephalon
intercourse: coitus, copulation
    See also sex act
intermittent: arrhythmic
intern: resident
intersex: hermaphrodite

interspace: interstice, lacuna, sulcus

intestine: enter-, entero-, alimentary canal, appendix, cecum, colon, duodenum, enteron, ileum (small), jejunum, rectum (large), splanchna, vermiformis, viscera

intestine, absence: anenterous

intestine, embryonic: enteromere

intestine, produced by: enterogenous

intestine, science of: enterology, gastroenterology

intestine, small: enteral, enteric, enteron, ileum

intestine, within: enteral

intestine antigen: enteroantigen

intestine bleeding: enterorrhagia, enterostaxis

intestine blood vessels, obstruction: enterangiemphraxis

intestine calculus: alvinolith, enterolith, enterolithiasis, splanchnolith, stercolith

intestine cell: enterocyte

intestine dilation: aerenterectasia, enterectasia, enteroparesis, meteorism, tympanites

intestine disease producing: enteropathogenesis

intestine diseases: Crohn's, dysentery, enterohydrocele, enteroidea, enteromycosis, enteromyiasis, enteropathy, stercoroma, torminia enterocyst

intestine displacement: enteroptosis, indigitation, intussusception, invagination

intestine enlargement: enterauxe, enteromegaly, megacolon

intestine enzyme: enteropeptidase

intestine examination: colonoscopy, enterography

intestine examination, instrument: endoscope, enteroscope

intestine excision: duodenectomy, enterectomy, enteroapokleisis

intestine fever: enteroidea

intestine fixation: enterohepatopexy, enteropexy

intestine fold: circular plica, Kerckring's folds

intestine gland: enteraden

intestine gland inflammation: enteradenitis

intestine hernia: enterocele, enterocystocele, enteroepiplocele, enterohepatocele, enterhydrocele

intestine hormone: enterocrinin, enterogastrone, enterokinin

intestine incision: enterocholecystotomy, enterotomy

intestine infections: bacillary dysentery, enterobiasis, enterosepsis, enterotoxism, giardiasis, oxyuriasis, shigellosis, viral
See also worm diseases

intestine inflammation: dysentery, endoenteritis, enteritis, enterocolitis, enterogastritis, enterohepatitis, enteroneuritis, enteronitis, gastroenteritis, necrotizing enteritis, necrotizing enterocolitis, seroenteritis

intestine injection: enteroclysis

intestine irrigation: enteroclysis

intestine mass: stercoroma

intestine microorganism: enteropathogen

intestine movement: diastalsis, enterocinesia, peristalsis

intestine muscle: myenteron

intestine narrowing: enterostenosis

intestine obstruction: enterostasis, ileus, splanchnemphraxis, volvulus

intestine opening: colostomy, enterostomy

intestine origin: enterogenous

intestine pain: enteralgia, enterodynia

intestine paralysis: enteroplegia

intestine prolapse: enteroptosis

intestine protrusion of: eventration

intestine puncture: enterocentesis

intestine rupture: enterorrhexis
intestine spasm: enterospasm
intestine specialist: gastroenterologist
intestine surgery: Billroth's operation,
  enteroanastomosis,
  enteroapokleisis, enterochirurgia,
  enterocholecystostomy,
  enterocolectomy, enterocolostomy,
  enterocystoplasty,
  enteroenterostomy, enterolysis,
  enteroplasty, enteroptychia,
  enteroptychy, enterostomy
intestine suture: enterorrhaphy
intestine toxicity: enterosepsis,
  enterotoxin
intestine tumors: enterocystoma,
  gastrinoma
intestine ulceration: enterelcosis
intestine wound closure: enterocleisis
into: intro-
intoxicants: alcohol, drug, narcotic,
  opiate, soporific
intoxicants, abnormal craving for:
  alcoholomania
intoxication: acute alcoholism,
  crapulent, poisoning
intrinsic: congenital, hereditary,
  inborn, inbred, innate, inherited
invalid: convalescent, hypochondria,
  malingerer, neurasthenic,
  valetudinarian
inversion: enstrophe, entropion
investigate: analyze, dissect, examine,
  probe, research, study
invigorating: analeptic, antasthenia
involuntary: autonomic,
  contravolitional
involuntary action: abulia
involuntary response: reflex
involution: catagenesis, infolding,
  intussusception, invagination,
  inversion, retroflexion, retroversion
inward: end-, endo-, eso-, afferent,
  entad, introversion
ion migration: phoresis
irate: delerious

iris: irido-
iris, absence of: aniridia
iris atrophy: iridoleptynsis
iris defect: coloboma, pseudocoloboma
iris disease: iridadenosis, iridauxesis,
  iridemia, iridodialysis, iridopathy
iris excision: corectomy, iridectomy
iris hernia: iridocele
iris incision: corotomy, iridotomy
iris inflammation: iridocyclitis,
  iridokeratitis, iritis
iris paralysis: iridoparalysis,
  iridoplegia
iris prolapse: iridoptosis
iris softening: iridomalacia
iris surgery: coreplasty,
  iridocystectomy, iridolysis
iris swelling: iridoncus
iron: ferr-, ferri-, ferro-, sidero-
iron affinity: siderophilous
iron deficiency: asiderosis, chlorosis,
  sideropenia
iron-forming: siderogenous
iron lung: Drinker respirator
irrational: dementia, raving
irregular: anomalo-, poikilo-,
  aberrant, abnormal, anomalous,
  asymmetric, bosselated, deviant,
  heteromorphous
irregularity: anomaly, constipation,
  malformation
irrigate: lavage
irritable colon: colitis
irritated: algetic, inflamed
irritating: algetic, amyctic, inflamed
isolation: culture, quarantine,
  sequestration
itch: paresthesia, pruritus, scabies
itch, ulceration from: psorelcosis
itching: odaxetic, pruritus
itching, preventive: antipruritic
itch mite: scabies
ivory-like: eburneous

J

jaundice: ictero-, Crigler-Najjar syndrome, Dubin-Johnson syndrome, flavedo, hyperbilirubinemia, icterus, pedicterus, urobilinicterus
jaundice, absence of: anicteric
jaundice, after: posticteric
jaundice causing: icterogenic
jaundice preventive: anti-icteric
jaw: gnathio-, mandible, maxillary
jaw, abnormal: brachygnathia, hypognathous, opisthognathism
jaw, absence: agnathia
jaw, large: macrognathia, pachygnathous
jaw abnormality: anisognathous
jaw bone: mandible, maxilla
jaw malformation: ageniocephaly, atelognathia, augnathus, otocephalus, synotia
jaw points: gnathion, gonion
jaw projection: prognathism
jaw spasm: ankylostoma, lockjaw, trismus
jaw surgery: gnathoplasty
jaw tumor: adamantinoma, ameloblastoma, epulis
jealousy, abnormal: zelotypia
jealousy, fear of: zelophobia
jejunum: jejuno-
jejunum inflammation: jejunitis, jejunoileitis, perijejunitis
jejunum surgery: jejunectomy, jejunostomy, jejunotomy
jellylike: gel, gelatinous, viscid
jerk: chorea, convulsion, palsy, paroxism, reflex, spasm, St. Vitus' dance, tremor, twitch
jerky: convulsive, spastic
jet lag: circadian rhythm, desynchronosis
jock itch: tinea cruris
jogger's heel: calcaneal spurs, fasciitis

jogger's red urine: hemoglobinuria
join: articulate
joined: zygo-, conjugate
join in seam: -rhaphy
joint: arthr-, arthro-, articul-, articulation, articulus, contilaginous, enarthrosis, fibrous, ginglymus, gliding, sutural, symphysis, syndesmosis, synovial
joint, air in: pneumarthrosis
joint, around: periarticular
joint, artificial: nearthrosis, neoarthrosis, prosthesis, pseudarthrosis
joint, away from: abarticular
joint, ball and socket: enarthrosis
joint, blood in: hemarthrosis
joint, fluid removed: arthrocentesis
joint, gliding: acromioclavicular, arthrodia
joint, lack of: inarticulate
joint, movable: abarthrosis, aparthrosis, diarthrosis
joint, new: stereoarthrolysis
joint, partly movable: amphiarthrosis, synchondrosis
joint, pus in: arthrempyesis, arthroempyesis, arthropyosis, pyarthrosis
joint amputation: disarticulation, exarticulation
joint aspiration: arthrocentesis
joint bleeding: arthrorrhagia, hemarthrosis
joint calculus: arthrolith
joint cartilage inflammation: arthrochondritis
joint cavity, abnormal growth: arthrophyte
joint deformity: arthrodysplasia, arthrogryposis, dysarthrosis, loxarthron
joint diseases: ankylosis, arthritides, arthrogryposis, arthrokatadysis, arthronosos, arthro-ophthalmopathy, arthropathia, arthropathy, arthrosis, chondrocalcinosis, clutton's,

Heberden nodes, hydrarthrosis,
osteoarthritis, pedarthrocace,
pseudogout
joint disintegration: arthrocace
joint dislocation: abarticulation
joint dissection: synosteotomy
joint edema: arthredema
joint examination: arthroendoscopy,
arthrography,
arthropneumorentgenography,
arthroscopy
joint excision: arthrectomy
joint fixation: ankylosis, arthrodesis,
arthrogryposis, arthrokleisis,
gomphosis, synarthrodia,
synarthrophysis, synarthrosis,
syndesis, synostosis
joint fluid, excessive: hydrathrosis
joint hinge: condylarthrosis,
diarthrosis, ginglymus
joint incision: arthrotomy
joint inflammation: amarthritis,
arthritis, arthrochondritis,
arthromeningitis, arthrosteitis,
arthrosynovitis, enarthritis,
holarthritis, osteoarthritis,
panarthritis, periarthritis,
polyarthritis, synovitis
joint looseness: arthrochalasis
joint measurement: arthrometry
joint measurement, instrument for:
arthrometer
joint movement: angular,
circumduction, gliding, rotation
joint movement, excessive: flail
join together: anastomosis, concretion,
fusion, parabiosis
joint pain: arthralgia, arthrodynia,
arthroneuralgia
joint replacement: arthroplasty
joint rigidity: acampsia, ankylosis,
arthrokatadysis, arthrokleisis,
Otto's disease
joints: multiarticular, polyarticular
joints, study of: arthrology,
arthropathology

joint sensibility: arthresthesia
joint stiffening: arthrosclerosis
joint surgery: arthroclasia,
arthroereisis, arthrolysis,
arthroplasty, arthrostomy,
arthroxesis
joint swelling: arthrocele,
arthrophyma, bunion, elaiopathy,
eleopathy
joint trauma: fracture, sprain, strain
joint treatment: oleoarthrosis
joint tumor: arthroncus
jowl: *See* jaw
jug-shaped: arytenoid
juice: fluid, liquid, secretion, succus
See also blood, lymph
jumpy: convulsive, spastic, tremor
juncture: confluence, joint
junk: heroin
justice, fear of: dikephobia
justification: rationalization
jut: protuberance
juvenile: adolescent, child, minor,
pubescent, teenager, youth
juvenile cell: blasto-, blast,
metamyelocyte
juxtapose: appose, match, pair

K

kala-azar: leishmaniasis
keeled chest: pectus carinatum
keel-shaped: carinate
keratolytics: alcloxa, aldioxa, benzoyl
peroxide, coal tar,
dibenzothiophene, isotrentinoin,
motretinide, pictorin diolamine,
resorcinol, salicylic acid, tretinoin
ketone: keto-
ketones, excessive: hyperketonuria,
ketonemia, ketonuria, ketosis,
ketosuria
kidney: nephr-, nephro-, bladder,
excretory system, nephric,
nephron, nephros, ren, renal,
renopathy, ureters, urethra

kidney, abnormal:
oligomeganephronia
kidney, absence: anephric,
anephrogenesis
kidney, around: circumrenal,
perinephric, perirenal
kidney, artificial: hemodialysis
kidney, hardening of: nephrosclerosis
kidney, near: adrenal
kidney, originating in: nephrogenic
kidney, study of: nephrology
kidney dilation: caliectasis,
hydronephrosis, nephrohydrosis,
nephrydrosis, pyelectasis,
uronephrosis
kidney disease: azotemia,
glomerulonephritis,
glomerulosclerosis, Goodpasture
syndrome, hydrohematonephrosis,
hydronephrosis,
hydropyonephrosis, nephredema,
nephremia, nephroangiosclerosis,
nephrocalcinosis, nephrolithiasis,
nephropathy, nephrophthisis,
nephropyosis, nephrosis,
nephrydrosis, pneumokidney,
polycystic, pyonephrolithiasis,
pyelonephrosis, pyelopathy, uremia,
urohematonephrosis,
uropyonephrosis, uropyoureter
kidney disease treatment: dialysis
kidney displacement: nephroptosis
kidney enlargement: nephrauxe,
nephrectasia, nephrohypertrophy,
nephromegaly
kidney examination: pyelography,
pyeloscopy, renography
kidney excision: calicectomy,
heminephrectomy, nephrectomy,
nephroureterectomy
kidney fixation: myonephropexy,
nephrocolopexy, nephropexy
kidney function, lack of:
nephroparalysis
kidney hardening: nephrosclerosis
kidney hemorrhage: nephrorrhagia

kidney hernia: nephrocele
kidney incision: nephrolithotomy,
nephrotomy, pyelotomy
kidney inflammation: colinephritis,
nephrapostasis, nephritis,
nephrocystitis, nephropyelitis,
paranephritis, perinephritis,
pyelitis, pyelocystitis,
pyelonephritis, pyonephritis
kidney inflammation preventive:
antinephritic
kidney measurement: pyelometry
kidney obstruction: nephremphraxia
kidney pain: nephralgia, nephrocolic
kidney prolapse: nephrocoloptosis,
nephroptosis
kidneys, between: interrenal
kidney-shaped: nephroid, renal,
reniform
kidney softening: nephromalacia
kidney specialist: nephrologist,
urologist
kidney stone: nephrolith, renal
calculus
kidney stone crusher: lithotripter
kidney surgery: nephrolysis,
nephrostomy, nephrotresis,
pelvilithotomy, pelviolithotomy,
pyelocystostomosis, pyelolithotomy,
pyeloplasty, pyeloplication,
pyelostomy, renipuncture
kidney suturing: nephrorrhapy
kidney tumors: adenocarcinoma of the
kidney, capsuloma, clear cell
carcinoma, epinephroma,
nephradenoma, nephroma,
nephroncus, renal cell carcinoma,
Wilms' tumor
kill: -cide, abortifacient, bactericide,
euthanasia, fungicide, germicide,
infanticide, insecticide, suicide
kink: cramp
kissing: osculation
kissing disease: infectious
mononucleosis
knee: gon-, genu, geniculum

knee, abnormal: gonycampsis
knee, back of: popliteal
knee, stiff: ankylosis
kneecap: patella, rotula, sesamoid bone
kneecap surgery: arthroscopy,
    patellapexy
knee cartilage: meniscus
knee cartilage removal: meniscetomy
knee disease: gonyocele, gonyoncus
knee inflammation: gonarthritis
knee ligaments: cruciate
kneelike: geniculum
knee pain: gonalgia
knee surgery: arthroplasty,
    gonarthrotomy, meniscectomy
knee tumor: gonatocele, gonyoncus
knife: -tome, lancet, scalpel
knife, large: scalprum
knifelike: lancinating, spatula
knives, fear of: aichmophobia
knob: nodule, papule, protuberance,
    tubercle, tumor
knock-knee: genu valgum,
    gonycrotesis, tragopodia
knock-out drops: chloral hydrate
knuckle: articulus

L

labor: taco-, accouchement, birth,
    childbirth, parturition, tocus
labor, abnormal: dystocia, parodynia
labor, before: antepartum
labor, changes in vagina: effacement
labor, difficult: dystocia
labor, dry: xerotocia
labor, rapid: oxytocia
labor assistant: accoucheur, midwife,
    monitrice, obstetrician
labor inducer: carboprost, dinoprost,
    dinoprostone, ecbolic, ergonovine,
    meteneprost, methylergonovine,
    oxytocin, quipazine, sparteine
labor inhibitors: isoxsuprine, ritodrine,
    terbutaline

labor pains: parodynia
labyrinth inflammation: labyrinthitis,
    perilabyrinthitis
laceration: cut, gash, lancination,
    mutilation, scratch, wound
lack: defect, deficiency
lacrimal duct calculus: dacryolith,
    dacryolithiasis
lacrimal duct discharge:
    dacryoblennorrhea
lacrimal duct disease: dacryopyorrhea
lacrimal duct excision:
    dacryocystectomy
lacrimal duct fistula: dacryosyrinx
lacrimal duct hernia: dacryocystocele
lacrimal duct incision:
    dacryocystotomy
lacrimal duct inflammation:
    dacryocanaliculitis, dacryocystitis,
    dacryocystoblennorrhea,
    dacryosolenitis
lacrimal duct obstruction:
    dacryagogatresia,
    dacryocystorhinostenosis,
    dacryocystostenosis, dacryostenosis
lacrimal duct pain: dacryocystalgia
lacrimal duct prolapse:
    dacryocystoptosis
lacrimal duct protrusion: dacryocele,
    dacryocystocele
lacrimal duct surgery:
    dacryocystorhinostomy,
    dacryocystostomy
lacrimal duct swelling: dacryoma
lacrimal duct ulceration: dacryohelcosis
lacrimal gland calculus: dacryolith
lacrimal gland induration:
    dacryadenoscirrhus
lacrimal gland inflammation:
    dacryadenitis, dacryoadenitis
lacrimal gland pain: dacryoadenalgia,
    dacryocystalgia
lacrimal gland tumor: dacryoma
lacrimal sac: dacryocyst
lactic acid in blood: lactacidemia,
    lacticemia

lactic acid in urine: lactaciduria
lactose in milk, excessive:
　saccharogalactorrhea
lacuna: cavity, fissure, interspace
Laetrile: amygdalin
lame: disabled, impaired
lameness: claudication
lamina: cortex, integument,
　membrane, skin
lamina inflammation: laminitis
laminate: desquamate, exfoliate
lancet: fleam, scalpel
language disorder: *See* speech
　disorders
languid: anemic, atonic, faint,
　inanimate, supine, valetudinarian,
　weak
languor: adynamia, asthenia, atony,
　debility, lethargy
lank: emaciated, gaunt
lapse: degenerate, deteriorate,
　recidivism, regression, relapse
large: macr-, macro-, mega-, vastus
large intestine: colon
large objects, fear of: megalophobia
large toe: hallux
larynx: laryngo-, arytenoid cartilage,
　cricoid cartilage, epiglottis, glottis,
　thyroid cartilage, vocal cords
larynx, air sac in: laryngocele
larynx, study of: laryngology
larynx bleeding: laryngorrhagia
larnyx closure: laryngospasm
larynx disease: laryngopathy
larynx dryness: laryngoxerosis
larynx examination: laryngoscopy
larynx examination instrument:
　laryngoscope
larynx excision: laryngectomy
larynx incision: laryngocentesis,
　laryngotomy
larynx inflammation: laryngitis,
　laryngopharyngitis, perilaryngitis
larynx narrowing: laryngostenosis
larynx paralysis: laryngoparalysis,
　laryngoplegia, logoplegia

larynx prolapse: laryngoptosis
larynx spasm: laryngismus,
　laryngospasm
larynx specialist: laryngologist
larynx surgery: laryngofissure,
　laryngoplasty
larynx swelling: laryngocele
last: caudad, posterior, terminal
latent: dormant, intermittent,
　potential
late-occurring: tardive
late onset: abiotrophy
later: sequential
latticelike: cancellous, reticular
laudanum: opium
laugh: risus
laugh, abnormal: risus sardonicus
laugh, inability to: aphonogelia
laughing gas: nitrous oxide
laughter, hysterical: cachinnation
law: nomo-, principle
laxative: aperient, aperitive, bisacodyl,
　bisoxatin, casanthranol, cascara,
　caster oil, cathartic, danthron,
　docusate, hydragogue, ipecac,
　lactulose, methylcellulose, milk of
　magnesia, mineral oil,
　oxyphenisatin, phenolphthalein,
　physic, poloxamer, polycarbophil,
　psyllium, purgative, senna,
　sennosides
layer: cortex, disk, integument,
　lamella, lamina, laryngismus,
　membrane, panniculus, stratum
layered: stratified, stratiform
laziness: inactivity, inertia, lethargy,
　somnolence, topor
lead: plumbum
leader: -agogue
lead poisoning: plumbism, saturnism
lead produced: saturnine
leak: aperature, cleft, defluxion,
　dehiscence, drain, effusion, fissure,
　incision, incontinent, orifice,
　puncture
lean: emaciated, gaunt

leaping: saltation
learning disability: attention defecit
disorder, dysgraphia, dyslexia,
hyperactivity, hyperkinesis,
minimal brain dysfunction
lechery: satyriasis
leech: annelid, Haemadipsa, Hirudo,
Limnatis, Macrobdella, Sanguisuga
leech infestation: hirudiniasis
leech killer: hirudicide
left: levo-, sinistro-, sinistra
left, fear of: levophobia
left-eared: sinistraural
left-eyed: sinistrocular,
sinistrocularity
left-footed: sinistropedal
left-handed: mancinism, sinistrality,
sinistromanual
left side, fear of: levophobia
left-turning: levogyrous, levorotatory,
levotorsion, sinistrogyration,
sinistrorse, sinistrotorsion
leftward: sinistrad
leg: crur-, appendage, calf, crus,
femur, fibula, limb, lower
extremity, patella, thigh, tibia
leg, abnormal number: polymelia,
polyscelia
leg, turned inward: pronation
leg, turned outward: supination
leg, wasting of: acnemia
legal: forensic
leg calf: sura
leg cramp: claudication, systremma
leg fracture: Gosselin's, Pott's, Stieda's
leg muscles: adductors, extensors,
gastrocnemius, gluteals, gracilis,
hamstrings, iliopsoas, peroneus,
piriformis, quadriceps, rectus,
sartorius, soleus, tibialis, vastus
leg pain: brachialgia, claudication,
sciatica, shin splints, skelalgia
leg paralysis: paraparesis, paraplectic,
paraplegia, quadraplegia
legs, absence of: acnemia
legs, fused: sirenomelia, symmelia,
sympodia, sympus

legs, large: macroscelia
legs, normal: mesoscelia
legs, short: microscelia
legs and arms: acral, extremities
leg swelling: bucnemia, elephantiasis,
phlegmasia alba dolens
lens: phaco-, bifocal, aplanatic,
apochromatic, eyeglass, monocle,
objective, ocular, pantoscopic,
planoconcave, planoconvex, trifocal
lens, abnormal: plesiopia
lens, absence: aphakia
lens, behind: retrolental
lens, small: microlentia, microphakia
lens dislocation: phacecele,
phacometachoresis, phacoplanesis
lens dissolution: phacoemulsification,
phacolysis, phakolysis
lens hardening: phacosclerosis
lens inflammation: crystalloiditis,
lentitis, phacitis, phacocystitis,
phacohymenitis
lens opacity: cataract, phacoscotasmus
lens protrusion: lenticonus
lens-shaped: lentiform, phacoid
lens softening: phacomalacia
lens surgery: phacocystectomy,
phacoerysis
leprosy: Hansen's disease
leprosy, study of: leprology
lesbian: homosexual, sapphism
lesion: abrasion, abscess, blister, boil,
bulla, chancre, contusion,
excoriation, laceration, pustule,
sore, trauma, ulcer, vesicle, wound
less: mio-
lethal: fatal, malignant, noxious, toxic
lethargy: cataphora, narcosis,
somnolence
letup: remission
leukocytes: *See* white blood cell
Leydig cells, absence of: aleydigism
lice: Pediculus, Pthirus
lice, fear of: pediculophobia
lice destroyer: pediculicide
lice infestation: pediculation,
pediculosis, phthiriasis

licentiousness: nymphomania,
    satyriasis
lid: cap, cover, operculum, stopper
    See also eyelid
lie detector: polygraph
lie down: clino-
lie face down: procumbent, prone,
    recumbent, ventricumbent
lie face up: supine
life: bio-, bios
life, against: antibiotic
life, science of: biology, bionomy,
    physiology
life destroying: biolytic
life functions: biotics
lifeless: abiosis, azoic
life prolongation: apothanasia
ligament: desmo-
ligament, abnormal: syndesmectopia
ligament disease: desmopathy
ligament excision: syndesmectomy
ligament fixation: syndesmopexy
ligament incision: desmotomy,
    syndesmotomy
ligament inflammation: desmitis,
    syndesmitis
ligament joined: syndesmopexy
ligament pain: desmalgia, desmodynia
ligament rupture: desmorrhexis
ligament stretching: desmectasia
ligament surgery: desmopyknosis,
    syndesmotomy, syndesmoplasty
ligament suturing: syndesmorrhaphy
light: phot-, photo-, photic, radiation
light, bent: refraction
light, broken up: diffraction
light, cold: chemiluminescence
light, fear of: astrapophobia,
    phengophobia, photangiophobia,
    photophobia
light, pain from: photalgia, photodynia
light, reaction to: chemotropism,
    galvanotropism, geotropism,
    photaxis, phototropism,
    rheotropism, stereotropism,
    thermotropism, tropism

light, sensation: centrophose, phose
light emission: bioluminescence,
    phosphorescence
light flashes: coruscation
light-headed: dizziness, giddiness,
    vertiginous.
light-induced diseases:
    photodermatitis, photoncia,
    photonosus, photopathy,
    photoretinitis, phototoxis
light-induced disintegration: photolysis
light-induced motion: photokinetic
light-induced sneezing:
    photoptarmosis, photo sneezing
light inducing: photogenic
lightning, fear of: astraphobia,
    keraunophobia, photophobia
light psychosis: photomania
light receptive: photoreceptor
light reflection: anaclasis
light refraction: anaclasis, dioptrics
light seeking: photophilic
light-sensitive cells: rods, cones
light sensitivity: photodysphoria,
    photesthesis, photosensitivity
light therapy: actinopraxis,
    chromotherapy, lucotherapy,
    phototherapy
like: analogous, homogeneous,
    homologous
like cures like: homeopathy
likeness: homeo-, homo-
limb: acro-, arm, extremity, leg,
    prosthesis
    See also extremity
limb, absence: acolous, amelia,
    dysmelia
limb, absence of feeling in:
    acroagnosis, acroanesthesia
limb, one: monomelic, monoplegia
limb, premature aging: acrogeria
limb, surgically removed: amputation
limb deformity:
    acrocephalosyndactylia, acromicria,
    Apert's syndrome, cacomelia,
    camptomelia, ectromelia,
    meromelia, peromelia, phocomelia

limb end: foot, hand, prosthesis, stump
limb feeling: acrognosis
limb fusion: sirenomelia, symmelia, sympodia, sympus
limb pain: melalgia, melagra
limb rigidity: acampsia
limbs, unequal: anisomelia
limb swelling: trophedema
lime: calx
limp: flaccid, lame
limping: claudication
line: boundary, commissure, linea, wrinkle
lineage: pedigree, progeny
liniment: balm, cerate, demulcent, emollient, lotion, unguent
liniment application: embrocation
link: interlacing, isthmus, nexus
lip: cheil-, -cheilia, cheilo-, chilo-, labio-, eclabium, labium, procheilon, prolabium
lip, cleft: cheiloschisis
lip, large: macrocheilia, macrolabia
lip, short: brachycheilia
lip, small: microcheilia
lip abnormality: atelocheilia, cheilognathopalatoschisis, cheiloschisis, harelip
lip diseases: ankylochilia, cheilosis, labiomycosis, syncheilia
lip dryness: xerocheilia
lip eversion: cheilectropion, chilectropion
lip examination: cheiloangioscopy
lip incision: cheilotomy
lip inflammation: cheilitis, perleche
lip pain: cheilalgia
lips, absence: acheilia
lips, thick: pachycheilia
lip surgery: cheiloplasty, cheilostomatoplasty, labioplasty
lip suturing: cheilorrhaphy
lip tumor: cheilocarcinoma
liquefaction: colliquation, deliquescence
liquid: decoction, fluid extract, infusion, juice, milk, oleoresin, tincture, water

liquid, absence: aneroid
liquid absorption: imbibition, insudation
liquid conversion: condense, dissolve, liquefaction, saturation
liquid deficiency: dehydration, desiccation, oligoposy
lisp: sibilate
listening: auscultation
listlessness: anergia, apathy, dormant, lethargy, torpid
litter: sling, stretcher
livable: viable
liver: hepat-, hepato-
liver, atrophied: hepatatrophia
liver, produced by: hepatogenic
liver, small: microhepatia
liver breath: fetor hepaticus
liver calculus: hepatolith
liver cell: hepatocyte
liver diseases: cirrhosis, clonorchiasis, Crigler-Najjar disease, Dubin-Johnson syndrome, Farre's tubercles, fascioliasis, Gilbert's syndrome, hepatopathy, Israels syndrome, opisthorchiasis, Rotor syndrome
liver enlargement: hepatauxe, hepatomegaly, megalohepatia
liver excision: hepatectomy
liver flap: asterixis
liver fluke: Clonorchis, Fasciola hepatica, Opisthorchis
liver hernia: hepatocele
liver incision: hepaticotomy
liver inflammation: hepatitis, parahepatitis, perihepatitis, purohepatitis, serohepatitis
liver pain: hepatalgia, hepatodynia
liver palpation: dipping
liver rupture: hepatorrhexis
liver specialist: hepatologist
liver spots: chloasma hepaticum, melasma
liver surgery: hepaticodochotomy, hepaticoenterostomy, hepaticogastrostomy, hepaticolithotomy, hepaticostomy

liver suturing: hepatorrhaphy
liver treatment: hepatotherapy
liver tumor: hepatoma
live together: cohabit, commensalism,
    metabiosis, mutualism, parasitism,
    symbiosis
livid: cyanotic
living: animate, organic, viable
living organism: bion
lobe: node, tubercle
lobe, surgery of: lobectomy, lobotomy
localized: in situ
locked in, fear of being:
    claustrophobia, clithrophobia
lockjaw: ankylostoma, tetanus,
    trismus
loin: lumbo-, lumbar, lumbus
loin muscle: psoas
loin pain: lumbago, osphyalgia,
    sciatica
long: dolicho-
longevity: life span, macrobiosis
long-lasting: chronic
loneliness, fear of: eremophobia
looked at, fear of being: scopophobia
loop: arc, convolution, helix,
    intrauterine device
looplike: anchylo-, ancylo-, anylo-,
    ansate, ansiform
loop structure: ansa
loose: lyo-, flaccid
lopsided: asymmetrical,
    disproportionate, unsymmetrical
loss of weight sense: abarognosis,
    baragnosis
loss of willpower: abulia
lotion: balm, cerate, collyrium,
    demulcent, emollient, lubricant,
    ointment, salve, unguent
loudness: amplitude, resonance, sone
loudness, of speech: stentorophonic
Lou Gehrig disease: amyotrophic
    lateral sclerosis
love: eroto-
love, self: autophilia, egomania,
    narcissism

love for: -philia
love potion: philter
low blood bicarbonate: acarbia
low blood pressure: hypotension
low temperature: hypothermia
lozenge: bolus, electuary, lincture,
    linctus, pastille, pill, rotula, tablet,
    troche, trochiscus
lubricant: emollient, ointment,
    unguent
lucid: crystalline, hyaline, pellucid,
    vitreous
lues: syphilis
lukewarm: tepid
lull: anesthetize, hypnotize,
    mesmerize, sedate, tranquilize
lumbar inflammation: osphyitis,
    osphyomelitis
lump: callus, carbuncle, condyle, corn,
    cyst, fibroma, gelosis, gibbus,
    myogelosis, neoplasm, node, nodule,
    tumescence, tumor, wart, wen
lump in throat: globus hystericus,
    spheresthesia
lumpy: grumose
lumpy jaw: actinomycosis
lunacy: dementia, insanity, mania,
    neurosis, psychosis
lunar caustic: silver nitrite
lung: pulmo-, pulmono-, bronchioles,
    bronchium, bronchus, carina
    See also bronchial, respiration
lung, absent: apulmonism
lung, iron: Drinker respirator
lung, membrane around: pleura
lung air pressure: bronchi-, broncho-,
    alveolus, bronchiole, bronchus
lung air removal: exhalation,
    exsufflation, respiration
lung bleeding: hemoptysis,
    pneumorrhagia
lung calculus: broncholith,
    pneumolithiasis
lung capacity determination:
    pulmometry, spirometry
lung collapse: apicolysis, atelectasis,
    pleuropneumonolysis, plombage,
    pneumothorax

lung collapse, congenital: anectasis
lung compression: oleothorax
lung diseases: adult respiratory
distress syndrome, aluminosis,
alveolar proteinosis,
anthracosilicosis, anthracosis,
apneumatosis, asbestosis, asthma,
atelectasis, bagassosis, bituminosis,
black lung, bronchitis, byssinosis,
chalicosis, chronic obstructive,
consolidation, emphysema,
empyema, farmer's lung,
Goodpasture syndrome,
granulomatosis, grinder's,
Hamman-Rich syndrome,
hemopneumothorax, hemosiderosis,
hemothorax, hydrothorax,
melanedema, pleurisy,
pneumoconiosis, pneumomelanosis,
pneumomycosis,
pneumonocirrhosis,
pneumonomycosis, pneumonopathy,
pneumonosis, siderosis, silicosis,
tuberculosis
lung examination: bronchography,
bronchoscopy, spirometry
lung examination instrument:
bronchoscope
lung excision: pneumonectomy,
pulmonectomy
lung fixation: pneumopexy,
pneumopleuroparietopexy
lung hernia: pneumatocele,
pneumocele, pneumonocele
lung incision: pneumonotomy
lung inflammation: alveobronchiolitis,
bronchopneumonia, interlobitis,
pneumonia, pneumonitis,
pneumopleuritis, pulmonitis
lung softening: pneumomalacia
lung sound, hollow: amphoric breath
sound
lung surgery: pneumolysis,
pneumonolysis
lung suturing: pneumonorrhaphy
lung treatment: pneumatotherapy

lust: acolasia, eroticism, libido
lying: mythomania
lying, pathologic: pseudologia,
pseudomania
lying down: clinostatism, decubation
lying face down: procumbent, prone,
recumbent, ventricumbent
lying face up: supine
lying in: confinement
lymph: lymph-, lympho-
lymph accumulation: lymphedema
lymphatic: humeral, ichorous,
inanimate, languid, lethargic,
phlegmatic, serous, sluggish, torpid
lymphatic disease: lymphopathy
lymphatic glands, enlarged: adenia
lymph discharge: lymphorrhagia,
lymphorrhea
lymph flow stoppage: lymphostasis
lymph formation: lymphogenesis
lymphlike: ichorus, lymphoid
lymph node diseases: Hodgkin's
disease, lymphadenopathy,
lymphosarcoma
lymph node enlargement:
adenolymphocele,
lymphadenhypertrophy,
lymphadenia, lymphadenoma,
lymphoma
lymph node excision:
lymphadenectomy,
lymphangiectomy
lymph node inflammation: adenia,
adenitis, adenolymphitis, bubo,
deradenitis, lymphadenitis
lymph node tuberculosis: scrofula
lymph node tumor: adenolymphoma,
deradenoncus
lymphocyte, large: macrolymphocyte
lymphocyte production:
lymphocytopoiesis, lymphopoiesis
lymphocytes, decreased:
lymphocytopenia, lymphopenia
lymphocytes, increased: achroacytosis,
lymphocythemia, lymphocytosis
lymphocytes, tumor of:
lymphoblastoma

lymphoid tissue, in urine: lymphuria
lymphoid tissue excision:
    lymphoidectomy
lymphoid tissue tumor: Burkitt's
    lymphoma, Hodgkin's disease,
    lymphoma, lymphosarcoma
lymphoma: Burkitt's, Hodgkin's
    disease
lymph vessel dilation:
    lymphangiectasis, lymphectasia
lymph vessel incision:
    lymphangiotomy
lymph vessel inflammation: angiitis,
    angioleukitis, angiolymphitis,
    lymphangiophlebitis, lymphangitis,
    perilymphangitis,
    thrombolymphangitis
lymph vessel obstruction: chyloderma,
    elephantiasis, lymphedema,
    myelolymphangioma,
    pachydermatosis
lymph vessel tumor: angiolymphoma,
    chylangioma, lymphadenoma,
    lymphangiofibroma,
    lymphangioma,
    lymphangiosarcoma,
    lymphendothelioma

M

machinery, fear of: mechanophobia
macula: comedo, nevus
mad: insane, mental disorder, rabid
magnification: amplification,
    enlargement, expansion
magnifier: lens, electron microscope,
    microscope
maidenhead: hymen
maim: disable, dismember, handicap,
    impair
malabsorption diseases: celiac, gluten
    enteropathy, sprue, steatorrhea,
    tropical sprue, Whipple's disease
    See also deficiency disease
malady: affliction, disability, disease,
    disorder, infection, mental
    disorder, wound

malaise: cenesthopathia
malaria: Plasmodium
malaria, after: postmalarial,
    postpaludal
malaria, study of: malariology
malaria therapy: antimalarial,
    antipaludian, chloroguanide,
    chloroquine
male: andr-, andro-, arrheno-
male, breast development:
    gynecomastia
male, breast milk secretion:
    androgalactozemia
male, castrated: eunuch
male, diseases of: andropathy
male, morbid dislike of: androphobia
male, sexless: castrate, eunuch
male, study of: andrology
male and female: androgyne, bisexual,
    gynander, gynandroid,
    gynandromorph, hermaphroditism,
    intersex, pseudohermaphroditism
male hormones: andosterone, andrin,
    androgen
male hormones, deficient:
    eunuchoidism
malelike: android, masculine, virile
males, aversion to: apandria,
    apanthropia
male sex cell: androcyte
male sex organs: epididymis, glans,
    penis, prepuce, prostate,
    seminiferous tubules, vas deferens
malformation: anomaly, birth defect,
    peronia
malignant: fatal, lethal, toxic, virulent
malingering: Munchausen syndrome
malnutrition: anorexia, athrepsia,
    atrophia, cacatrophy, cachexia,
    denutrition, marasmus
malodorous: putrescent, putrid, rancid
malpositioned: displacement, dystopia,
    ectopia
Malta fever: brucellosis
mammary gland: See breast
man: andr-, andro-, anthropo-,
    android, Homo sapiens, male

man, fear of: androphobia
man, study of: anthropology
mange: exanthema, psoriasis, scabies
maniacal: delirious, frenetic, hysterical
manias: ablulomania, agromania,
    amenomania, aphrodisiomania,
    arithmomania, bromomania,
    bruxomania, brychomania,
    callomania, camphoromania,
    chaeromania, choreomania,
    choromania, cocainomania,
    dacnomania, demonomania,
    dipsomania, drapetomania,
    dromomania, egomania,
    enosimania, ergasiomania,
    erotomania, fanaticism, impulsive
    obsession, kleptomania,
    megalomania, monomania,
    narcomania, necromania,
    nymphomania, oniomania,
    onomatomania, onychotillomania,
    opiomania, opsomania, oreximania,
    parateresiomania, peotillomania,
    phagomania, pharmacomania,
    photomania, phonomania,
    planomania, plutomania,
    poriomania, posiomania,
    potomania, pseudomania,
    pyromania, sebastomania,
    sitiomania, sitomania,
    symmetromania, syphilomania,
    theomania, tomomania,
    toxicomania, trichokryptomania,
    trichorrhexomania,
    trichotillomania, tristimania,
    tromomania, verbomania, zoomania
manic: hyperactive, hyperphrenic
manic-depressive disease: bipolar
    disorder
manifest: palpable, phanic
manipulation: encheiresis
manipulation, therapeutic:
    chiropractic, naprapathy, medical
    orthopedist
many: multi-, poly-
marble bones: Albers-Schoenberg
    disease, osteopetrosis

margin: border, edge, ora, rim
mark: nevus
marriage, fear of: gamophobia
marriage aversion: misogamy
marrow: medulla
    See also bone marrow
marrow inflammation: medullitis,
    medulloarthritis, myelitis
marrowlike: myeloid
marsh fever: malaria
masculine: virile
masculine appearance: andromorphous
mass: -blastema, onco-, bolus, bulb,
    caruncle, conglobate, corpus, cyst,
    tumor
massage: anatripsis, chirismus,
    clapping, effeurage,
    electromassage, flagellation,
    foulage, friction, frolement,
    frottage, fustigation, gelotripsy,
    hachement, hydromassage,
    kneeding, malaxation, petrissage,
    pincement,
    pneumothermomassage,
    pointillage, sciage, seismotherapy
    sismotherapy, shaking, stroke,
    Swedish, tapotement
    thermomassage, vibration,
    vibromassage
mastication difficulty: amasesis,
    dysmasesis
mastoid excision: mastoidectomy
mastoid inflammation:
    intramastoiditis, mastoiditis
mastoid surgery: mastoidotomy
masturbation, abnormality:
    mentulomania, peotillomania,
    pseudomasturbation, psycholagny
materialism, fear of: hylephobia
mating: copulation, incest
    See also sex act
matter: gleet, ichor, leukorrhea,
    mucus, phlegm, plasma,
    protoplasm, purulence, pus, sanies,
    suppuration
matter, conversion of: anabolism,
    catabolism

maturation: growth, ripening
maxilla inflammation: maxillitis
maxillary sinus inflammation:
    siagonantritis
maxilla tumor: adenomeloblastoma
meal, after: postprandial
meal, before: preprandial
measles: black, Koplik's spots, morbilli,
    rubella, rubeola
measleslike: morbilliform
measure: -metry
meat, fear of: carnophobia
mechanical devices: brace, crutch,
    orthotics, wheelchair
mediastinum inflammation:
    mediastinitis
medical anatomy: anatomicomedical
medical geography: geomedicine,
    nosochthonography, nosogeography
medical history: anamnesis,
    catamnesis, follow-up
medical science: iatrology
medical symbol: caduceus, staff of
    Aesculapius
medical treatment: acupuncture,
    allopathy, homeopathy,
    pharmacognosy, surgery,
    therapeutics
medication, applied by rubbing:
    anatriptic, ointment, salve
medicinals: ampule, apozem, bolus,
    capsule, cerate, confection,
    decoction, demulcent, electuary,
    elixir, embrocation, emollient,
    extract, lamella, lenitive, liniment,
    lotion, lozenge, magma, mistura,
    mixture, ointment, pill, plaster,
    potion, powder, prescription, rotula,
    suppository, tabella, tablet,
    tincture, tonic, troche, trochiscus,
    unguent, wafer
medicine: antibiotic, antitoxin,
    armamentarium, drug, materia
    medica, medicament, medication,
    medicinals, pharmaceutical,
    preparation, prescription, vaccine

medicine, dosage: posology
medicine, in vein: intravenous,
    phleboclysis, venoclysis
medicine, multiuse: polychrest
medicine, through skin: endermatic,
    endermosis, transdermal
medicine container: ampule, cachet,
    capsule, phial, syringe, vial
medicines, fear of: pharmacophobia
Mediterranean anemia: Cooley's
    anemia, thalassemia
Mediterranean fever: brucellosis,
    polyserositis
medulla oblongata disease:
    syringobulbia, syringomelia
medullary: See neural
meibomian gland inflammation:
    adenophthalmia, blepharadenitis
melancholy: acedia, depression,
    oligoria, tristimania
melanin formation: melanogenesis
meld: synthesize
member: limb, organ, penis
membrane: meningo-
membrane, weblike: patagium,
    pterygium
membrane layer: panniculus
membranes: albuginea, allantois,
    amniochorion, amnion, anal,
    arachnoid, axilemma, axolemma,
    basement, Bichat's, Bruch's,
    Brunn's, buconasal,
    bucopharyngeal, capsule, cell,
    chorion, cloacal, conjunctiva,
    cutaneous, decidua, Descemet's,
    dura mater, elastic, enamel,
    endocardium, endocranium,
    endometrium, endorrhachis,
    endosterum, ependyma,
    epicapillary, exocelomic, false,
    fascia, fetal, glassy, hyaline,
    hymen, hypoglossal, intercostal,
    Jackson's, leptomeninges,
    meninges, mucous, nictitating,
    obturator, olfactory, Payr's,
    pericardium, perichondrium,
    pericranium, peridesmium,
    periostium, peritoneum,
    piarachnoid, pileum, placental,

plasma, pleura, postsynaptic,
presynaptic, retinaculum,
sarcolemma, schneiderian, serosa,
serous, synaptolemma, synovial,
telolemma, testis, Tourtual's,
transversalis, tunica, tympanic,
velamen, velamentum, vitreus,
Wachendorf's, Zinn's
membranes, false: neohyman,
neomembrane, pseudomembrane
membranes, science of: hymenology
memory: -mnesia, -mnestic, affect,
anamnesis, hypermnesia,
kinesthetic, long-term, mnemonic,
recall, screen, short-term, visual
memory, abnormal: anomia,
anterograde, dysmnesia, ecmnesia,
hypomnesia, paramnesia,
pseudomnesia
memory, poor: mnemasthenia
memory, subconscious:
cryptanamnesia, cryptomnesia
memory device: mnemonics
memory disorders: Alzheimer's
disease, Creutzfeldt-Jacob disease,
dementias, Hungtington's disease,
Korsakoff's syndrome, obstructive
hydrocephalus, Pick's disease,
Wilson's disease
memory loss: acousmatamnesia,
amnesia, hysterical, lethe,
lethologica, post-traumatic,
retrograde
men, bad, fear of: pavor scleris,
scelerophobia
men, fear of: androphobia
mend: convalesce, recuperate,
rehabilitate, repair
meninges: dura mater, arachnoid, pia
mater; leptomeninges
meninges bleeding: meningorrhagia,
meningorrhea
meninges disease: meningioma,
meningism, meningocele,
meningopathy
meninges hernia: meningocele,
meningoencephalocele,
meningomyelocele

meninges inflammation:
cephalomeningitis, meningitis,
meningoencephalitis
meninges tumor: meningioma
meningitis, fear of: meningitophobia
menses: meno-
menstrual cramps: dysmenorrhea
menstruation: catamenia, emmenia,
menacme, menarine, menorrhea,
menses, monophania
menstruation, abnormal: amenia,
cephalomenia, cryptomenorrhea,
emmeniopathhy, hypermenorrhea,
hypomenorrhea, menhidrosis,
menometorrhagia, menoplania,
menorrhagia, menostasis,
menostaxis, menothermal,
menoxenia, myelomenia,
oligohypermenorrhea,
oligohypomenorrhea,
oligomenorrhea, paramenia,
polyhypermenorrhea,
polyhypomenorrhea,
polymenorrhea, xenomenia
menstruation, absence: amenorrhea,
menopause, menoschesis
menstruation, painful: algomenorrhea,
dysmenorrhea, menorrhalgia
menstruation inducer: emmenagogue,
hemagogue
menstruation odor: bromomenorrhea
mental: cognitive, cerebral, intellect,
intellectual, IQ, noesis, perception,
phrenic, psychical, psychological,
rational, reasoning, subconscious,
subliminal, thought
mental activity, measurement:
psychodometry
mental activity, rapid: tachyphrenia
mental diseases: -phrenia, affective
disorder, alcoholic psychosis,
algopsycholia, amenomania,
amentia, anergasia, anxiety
neurosis, aphrenia, aphronesia,
autism, autopsychosis, bipolar,
cacodemonia, catalepsy,
cataphrenia, catatonia,
chaeromania, compulsion,
conversion disorder, cynanthropy,

delirium, delirium tremens,
delusion, dementia,
depersonalization disorder,
depression, dipsomania,
dissociative, egomania, folie,
general paresis, hallucination,
hysteria, insanity, Korsakoff's
psychosis, lycanthropy, mania,
megalomania, melancholia,
monomania, multiple personality,
narcissism, neuroses, obsession,
obsessive-compulsive, oniomania,
onomatomania, opiomania,
oreximania, organic brain
syndrome, paralepsy, paranoia,
paraphora, parapraxia,
paratereseomania, parathymia,
peotillomania, perichareia,
phagomania, phantasmatormoria,
pharmacomania, phonomania,
photomania, phrenalgia,
phrenoplegia, planomania,
plutomania, poriomania,
posiomania, potomania,
pseudodementia, pseudomania,
psycholepsy, psycholgia,
psychoneurosis, psychoparesis,
psychopathy, psychorhythmia,
psychorrhea, psychosexual disorder,
psychosis, pyromania,
pyroptothymia, rhembasmus,
schizophrenia, senile dementia,
senile psychosis, somatoform
disorder
mental disease, drugs for:
antidepressant, antipsychotic,
neuroleptic, psychopharmacology,
psychotropic, tranquilizers
mental disease, religious:
sebastomania, theomania
mental disease, study of: psychiatry,
psychoanalysis, psychobiology,
psychology, psychopathology,
psychotherapy
mental disease, surgery for: lobotomy,
psychosurgery

mental disease specialist: alienist,
psychiatrist, psychoanalyst,
psychologist, therapist
mental feeling: affect, emotion
mental functioning, defective:
aphronia
mental hygiene: psychophylaxis
mental retardation: acataleptic,
amentia, aponoia, cephalonia,
Coffin-Siris syndrome, Down's
syndrome, feebleminded, Hunter's
syndrome, Hurler's syndrome,
hypophrenia, idiot, imbecile,
infantilism, moron, oligergasia,
oligophrenia, phenylketonuria,
Sandhoff's disease, Tay-Sachs
disease
mental state, normal: eunoia
mental suggestion: neuroinduction
mental tests: intelligence quotient,
personality, psychological,
psychometry
mercury poisoning: Minamata disease
mercy killing: euthanasia
mesentary inflammation: mesenteritis
mesentary surgery: mesenteriopexy,
mesenteriorrhaphy,
mesenteriplication, mesopexy,
mesorrhaphy
meshed: network, reticular
meshlike: texiform
mesmerism: anochlesia, catalepsy,
hypnosis, hypnotism
metabolism, breakdown: catabolism
metabolism, constructive: anabolism
metabolism, rapid: tachytrophism
metabolism diseases: albinism,
alkaptonuria,
argenosuccinicaciduria,
citrullinemia, cystathioninuria,
Dubin-Johnson syndrome,
Dyggve-Melchoir-Clausen
dysplasia, dysbolism, Forbes
disease, galactosemia, gout,
Hartnup disease, hemochromatosis,
histidinemia, Hunter's syndrome,
hypervalemia, hypophosphatasia,
Lesch-Nyhan syndrome,
lipodystrophy, oxalosis, pentosuria,

phenylketonuria, tyrosinemia,
tyrosinosis
See also glycogen storage diseases
metal, mixture of: alloy, amalgam
metals, fear of: metallophobia
metals, therapy with: metallotherapy,
siderism
metamorphosis: metaplasia,
metastasis, mutation,
transformation
metatarsal pain: metatarsalgia
metatarsal surgery: metatarsectomy
meteors, fear of: metearophobia
method: classification, maneuver,
technique, treatment
mice, fear of: musophobia
Mickey Finn: chloral hydrate
microorganism: bacteria, fungus,
helminth, mold, protozoa,
rickettsia, virus, yeasts
microorganism, live without oxygen:
anaerobe
microorganism, live with oxygen:
aerobe
microorganism preventive:
antibacterial, antimicrobial,
antiseptic, antitoxin
microwave treatment: diathermy
midbrain: mesencephalon
middle: medi-, medio-, meso-, medial,
mesad, mesiad, solar plexus
midline, toward: admedian
midriff: diaphragm
midwife: accoucheuse
migration: -phoresis, diapedesis,
diapiresis
mildew: blight, fungus, mold
milk: lact-, lacto-, breast, lac
milk, first after parturition: colostrum,
neogala
milk, lack of: agalactia, oligogalactia
milk, pressed from breast: expression
milk, produce: galactophorous,
lactigenous
milk cyst: galactocele, lactocele
milk diet: lactotherapy

milk duct: galactophore
milk duct inflammation:
galactophoritis
milk fever: galactopyra
milk flow, excessive: galactorrhea,
hypergalactia, hyperlactation,
lactorrhea, polygalactia,
superlactation
milk flow inducer: galactagogue,
galactopoietic, lactogen
milk flow suppression: agalorrhea,
antigalactagogue, antigalactic,
galactischia, galactophygous,
galactostasis, ischogalactic,
lactifuge
milk leg: phlegmasia cerulea dolens,
thrombosis
milk poisoning: tyrotoxism
milkpox: alastrim, amaas, variola
minor
milk protein: casein
milk secretion: galactosis, lactation,
lactiferous
milk secretion, in males:
androgalactozemia
milk secretion disorder: dysgalactia
milk sugar: lactose
milk teeth: deciduous
milk toxin: galactototoxicon,
galactoxin, lactotoxin
milky: lacteal, lactescent, lactic
milky ascites: chylous ascites
mimicry: mimesis
mind: ment-, phren-, phreno-, psych-,
psycho-, cerebral, cerebrum,
cognitive function, conscious, ego,
intellect, phronema, psyche,
subconscious
mind, fear of: psychophobia
mind, normal: phronesis, rational,
sane, sanity
mind, originating in: psychogenic
mind, state of: affect, mood
mind and body: psychophysiologic,
psychosomatic
mineral loss: demineralization

miner's lung: anthracosis
minute: atomic, dwarf, microscopic,
    nanoid, pygmy
mirrors, fear of: catoptrophobia,
    eisoptrophobia, spectrophobia
miscarriage: abortion
misinterpretation, fear of:
    symbolophobia
mismatched: incompatible,
    uncomplementary
misshapen: aberration, abnormality,
    anomaly, deformity, kyphosis,
    lordosis, malformation, monster
missiles, fear of: ballistophobia
mistreat: abuse, batter, injure, molest
mite: acaro-, acarid, Acarus, Pyemotes
mite, dread of: acarophobia
mite, study of: acarology
mite infestation: acariasis,
    trombiculosis
mix: amalgamate, coalesce, compound,
    crossbreed, cross-fertilize,
    homogenize, hybrid, interbreed,
    misce, synthesize
mixable: miscible
mixture: alloy, amalgam, assimilation,
    compound, concoction, hybrid
mobile: kinetic, motile
model: moulage, pattern, prototype
model case: index case, proband,
    propositus
moist: aqueous, modescent
moistening: humectant
moisture: hygro-
moisture, fear of: hygrophobia
moisture absorption: bibulous,
    hydrophiblous, hygroscopic
mold: blight, fungus, pattern,
    prototype, template
moldlike: mycelioid, mycoid
moldy: decaying, mucoriferous
mole: hydatid, macula, melanoma,
    nevus, spiloma, verruca, wart
molest: abuse, batter, injure, maltreat
money, fear of: chrematophobia
mongolism: Down's syndrome, trisomy
    G syndrome, trisomy 21

monilia: Candida
monilia infection: candidiasis,
    candidosis
monocytes, excessive: monocytosis
monocytes, reduced: monocytopenia
monsters: terato-, abrachiocephalus,
    acardius, acephalobrachius,
    acephalochirus, acephalogaster,
    acephalopodius, acephalostomus,
    acephalotharus, acephalus,
    acranius, anadidymus,
    anakatadidymus, celosomus,
    cephalothoracopagus, cyclocephalus,
    cyclopia, emmenic, endocymic,
    katadidymus, opodidymus,
    polysomatous, sirenomelus, sympus,
    teras, teratism, tricephalus,
    triocephalus, triophthalmos,
    triopodymus
monsters, study of: teratology
mood changes: psycholeptsy
moon-struck: delirious, frenzied,
    hysterical, maniacal
morbid: contaminated, degenerative,
    depressed, diseased, melancholia,
    pathogenic, phthisis
more: pleio-, pleo-, plio-, pluri-,
    adjunct
morgue: mortuary
morning sickness: hyperemesis
    gravidarum
moron: deficient, idiot, imbecile,
    mentally retarded
morphine-caused disorder:
    morphinism, morphinomania
mortal: lethal
mortality, study of: necrology
mortify: decompose, fester, gangrene,
    necrose, putrescent, suppurate
mosquito: Aedes, Haemagogus
mother: maternal, maternity, nurture,
    parent, procreate
mother's mark: birthmark, nevus
mother's milk: breast milk
motility, excessive: hyperkinesia,
    supermotility

motion: cine-, kine-, kinetic, motor
motion, fear of: kinesophobia
motion, loss of: paralysis
motion, science of: biomechanics,
  kinematics, kinesiology, kinetics
motionlessness: akinesia, dormant
motion sickness: air sickness, car
  sickness, kinectosis, kinesia,
  kinetosis, seasickness
motor abnormality: parakinesia
motor paralysis: anesthekinesia
motor slowness: bradykinesis
mountain fever: brucellosis, Colorado
  tick fever, Rocky Mountain spotted
  fever
mountain sickness: Acosta's disease,
  altitude sickness, hypsonosus,
  static, veta
mourn: grief
mouth: oro-, stomato-, buccal cavity,
  fauces, oral cavity, orifice, os
mouth, absence: aglossostomia,
  astomia, lipostomy
mouth, around: circumoral, perioral
mouth, gangrenous: cancrum oris,
  noma gangrenous
mouth, science of: stomatology
mouth, small: microstomia
mouth, softening: stomatomalacia
mouth, through: perlingual, peroral,
  per os
mouth, toward: adoral
mouth, wide: macrostomia
mouth accumulations: rhyparia,
  saburra, sordes
mouth bleeding: stomatorrhagia
mouth defect: atelostomia
mouth diseases: antitrismus,
  leukoplakia, Ludwig's angina,
  stomatomycosis, stomatopathy,
  stomatosis
mouth disease, study of: oralogy,
  stomatology
mouth dryness: xerostomia
mouth inflammation: stomatitis,
  thrush

mouth narrowing: stenostomia
mouth pain: stomatalgia,
  stomatodynia
mouth roof: palate, uraniscus
mouths, multiple: polystomatous
mouth sore: enanthema
mouth surgery: stomatoplasty
mouth-to-mouth resuscitation:
  cardiopulmonary resuscitation
mouth ulcers: aphthae
move, inability to: akinesia
move forward: anterograde
movement: cine-, kine-, kinesio-,
  mot-, defecation, diadochokinesia,
  excretion, kinesis, pronation,
  propalinal, supination
movement, away from: abduct
movement, backward: palinal,
  retrocedent, retrocession,
  retrograde
movement, circular: circumduction
movement, excessive: acrocinesia,
  hyperanakinesia, hyperkinesia,
  hypermotility
movement, fear of: kinesophobia
movement, involuntary: allokinesis,
  athetosis, syncinesis, synkinesis
movement, lack of: hypokinesia
movement, normal: eukinesia,
  eupraxia
movement, slow: bradykinesia
movement, toward: adduct, adient,
  afferent
movement, voluntary: autocinesia,
  autokinesia
movement abnormality: incoordination
movement disorders: amnestic
  apraxia, apraxia, ataxia, cataplexy,
  dysdiadochokinesia, dyskinesia,
  dyssynergia, hypometria,
  kinanesthesia, kinesioneurosis,
  tardive dyskinesia
movement disorder therapy:
  amantadine, benztropine,
  biperiden, bromocriptine,
  diphenhydramine, ethopropazine,
  levodopa, procyclidine,
  trihexyphenidyl

movement of joint: angular,
circumduction, gliding, rotation
movement of particles: diffusion,
diapedesis
movement perception: kinesthesia
movement therapy: kinesiatrics,
kinesiotherapy, kinesitherapy,
kinetotherapy
moxibustion: byssocausis
mucin in blood: mucinemia, myxemia
mucin in urine: mucinuria
mucosa removal: demucosation
mucus: blenn-, blenno-, myx-, myxo-,
phlegm
mucus, excessive: polyblennia
mucus, lack of: amyxia, amyxorrhea,
hypomyxia
mucus, vomiting: blennemesis
mucus and pus: mucopurulent
mucus cell: chalice cell, goblet cell
mucus cyst: mucocele, polypus
mucus discharge: apophlegmatic,
blennorrhagia, blennorrhea,
expectorant, myxorrhea
mucus discharge cessation:
blennostasis, blennostatic
mucus dissolving: mucolytic
mucus gland defect: myxasthenia
mucus gland inflammation:
blennadenitis, myxadenitis,
myxangitis
mucus gland tumor: myxadenoma,
myxoma
mucus in lung: blennothorax
mucus in urine: blennuria
mucus in vagina: mucocolpos
mucuslike: mucoid
mucus membrane ulceration: cancrum
oris, gangrenous stomatitis, noma
mucus producing: muciferous,
mucigenous, muciparous
mucus secreting: blennogenic,
muciferous
multi: poly-
multicolored: polychromatic
multifoci: polynesic

multiform: polymorphism
multinuclear: polykaryocyte,
polynuclear
multiple personality: dissociative
disorder
multiply: duplicate, generate, meiosis,
mitosis, propagate, replicate,
reproduce
mummified: papyraceous
mumps: epidemic parotitis, parotitis
murderous: hemothymia, phonomania
murmur: Austin-Flint, bruit,
fremitus, Graham Steel, susurrus,
thrill
muscle: my-, myo-, agonist,
antagonist, cardiac, smooth,
striated
See also movement
muscle, failure to develop: amyoplasia
muscle, failure to relax: achalasia,
cardiospasm
muscle, flabby: amyotonia,
dysmyotonia, dystonia, myotonia,
myotony
muscle, inability to move: akinesia
muscle, lack of tone: amyotonia
muscle, opposed by another muscle:
agonist, antagonist
muscle, originating in: myogenic
muscle, restless: akathisia
muscle, study of: electromyography,
myography, myology
muscle adhesion: myosynizesis
muscle atrophy: Aran-Duchenne
disease
muscle attachment: insertion, origin
muscle auscultation: dynamoscopy
muscle cell: myocyte, myoplasm,
sarcoplasm
muscle contractility: myotility
muscle contractions: chorea,
Sydenham's chorea
muscle control: dirigomotor
muscle coordination, abnormal: ataxia,
dystaxia, pseudoataxia
muscle degeneration: myocerosis,
myodemia, myodystrophy

muscle development, abnormal:
hypermyotrophy
muscle diseases: akinesia, apraxia,
Bell's palsy, cerebral palsy,
Charcot-Marie-Tooth disease,
dyspraxia, floppy infant syndrome,
Guillain-Barre syndrome,
Kugelberg-Welander disease,
Legg-Calve-Perthes disease,
muscular dystrophy, myasthenia
gravis, myodystrophy, myofibrosis,
myogelosis, myoischemia, myolysis,
myonecrosis, myoneurasthenia,
myonosus, myopathy, myosclerosis,
poliomyelitis, polyneuritis,
progressive neuropathic muscular
atrophy, trophotonus, Werdnig-
Hoffmann disease
muscle excision: myectomy
muscle fatigue: copodyskinesia
muscle fiber: myofibril
muscle force: inotropic, myodynamia
muscle formation: myogenetic,
myogenic
muscle formation, lack of: amyoplasia
muscle incision: myotomy
muscle inflammation: initis, myitis,
myocelitis, muocolpitis, myofascitis,
myositis, myotenositis,
perimyositis, sarcitis
muscle injury: strain
musclelike: myoid
muscle movement: clonus, myokinesis
muscle pain: kinesalgia, kinesialgia,
myalgia, myocelialgia, myodynia,
myosalgia
muscle paralysis: myoparalysis,
myoparesis
muscle power, diminished: adynamia,
hypodynamia
muscle producing: myogenic
muscle protein: actin, actinin, myosin
muscle relaxants: carisoprodol,
chlorphenesin, chlorzoxazone,
cyclobenzaprine, diazepam,
metaxalone, methocarbamol,
orphenadrine

muscle rupture: myodiastasis,
myorrhexia
muscle sheath: epimysium,
perimysium, sarcolemma
muscle shortening: contraction
muscle softening: myomalacia
muscle sound recording:
phonomyogram
muscle spasm: emprosthotonos,
kymatism, low back syndrome,
myoclonus, myoclonus multiplex,
myokymia, myopalmus, myospasm,
myotonus, opisthotonos, orthotonos,
paramyoclonus multiplex,
pleurothotonos, polymyoclonus,
strained back, synclonus,
Thomsen's disease, torticollis,
tortipelvis, vellication
muscle stretching: myotasis
muscle surgery: myomectomy,
myoplasty, myorrhaphy,
myotenontoplasty, myotenotomy,
myotonia, prorrhaphy
muscle tissue, deficient: amyous
muscle tone, lack of: atony
muscle tremor: amyostasia
muscle tumors: adenoleiomyofibroma,
myoblastoma, myocytoma,
myofibroma, myolipoma, myoma,
myosarcoma, myosteoma,
rhabdomyoma, rhabdomyosarcoma
muscle wasting: amyotrophic lateral
sclerosis, amyotrophy, myoatrophy
muscle weakness: amyosthenia,
myasthenia
musculoskeletal system, science of:
orthopedica
mushroom-shaped: fungiform
mustard plaster: sinapism
mute: aphonia, deaf-mute
mutilate: amputate, deformity,
dismember, dissection
mutter, delusional: mussitation
myelin destruction: demyelinate,
myelinolysis
myelin producing: myelinization,
myelinogenetic, myelinosis

myoglobin, in urine: myoglobinurea
myopia correction: myoporthosis
myosin, in urine: myosuria
myths, fear of: mythophobia

N

nail: onych-, onycho-, cuticle,
    fingernail, keratin, onyx, toenail,
    unguis
nail, abnormal: onychoheterotopia,
    paronychosis
nail, ingrown: acronyx,
    onychocryptosis, onyxis
nail atrophy: onchatrophia
nailbed: hyponychium, matrix unguis
nailbed inflammation: onychia,
    onychitis, onyxitis, paronychia,
    perionychia, perionyxis
nailbed overgrowth: onychauxis,
    onychogryposis
nail biting: onychophagy
nail breaking: onychoclasis
nail discoloration: azure lunulae
nail diseases: koilonychia,
    onychomycosis, onycho-
    osteodysplasia, onychopathy,
    onychophosis, onychophyma,
    onychoptosis, onychorrhexis,
    onychosis, paronychomycosis,
    Wardrop's disease
nail excision: onychectomy
nail hardening: scleronychia
nail incision: onychotomy
naillike: onychoid, ungual
nail malformation: onychodystrophy
nail producing: oncychogenic
nail root covering: cuticle, eponychium
nails, absent: anonychia
nails, black: melanonychia
nails, excessive growth: hyperonychia,
    megalonychosis
nails, picking at: onychotillomania
nails, soft: hapalonychia,
    onychomalacia

nails, thick: pachyonychia
nails, white spots in: canities unguium,
    leukonychia
nail separation: onycholysis
nail shedding: piptonychia
nail skinfold: vallum unguis
nail softening: onychomalacia
nail splitting: onychoschizia,
    schizonychia
nail tumor: onychoma
nail wall: vallum unguis
nail white: lunula
naked: nudo-, nude
nakedness, fear of: gymnophobia
nameless: innominate
names, fear of: onomatophobia
nape: nucha
narcissistic: autophilia, egomania
narcotic: amphetamine, analgesic,
    anodyne, antidepressant,
    belladonna, hallucinogen, hypnotic,
    morphine, opium, sedative,
    soporific, tranquilizer
narcotic craving: narcomania
narrow: lepto-, steno-
narrow head: stenobregmatic,
    stenocephaly
narrowing: coarctation, constriction,
    stenosis, stricture
narrow opening: stenopeic
nasal congestion: coryza, endorhinitis,
    pollinosis, rhinitis
nascent: embryonic
natural: physico-, physio-, inborn,
    inbred, innate
natural opiates: endorphins,
    enkephalin
nature of: -aceus
nausea: motion sickness, sicchasia
nausea preventive: antemetic,
    antiemetic, antinauseant,
    benzquinamide, buclizine,
    chlorpromazine, cyclizine,
    dimenhydramine, diphenidol,
    domperidone, dronabinol,
    flumeridone, haloperidol, meclizine,
    metocloperazine, metopimazine,
    perphenazine, prochlorperazine,

promethazine, scopolamine,
thiethylperazine, triflupromazine,
trimethobenzamide
nausea producing: nauseant
navel: omphal-, omphalo-, omphalos-,
omphalic, omphalus, umbilicus
navel, near: paraumbilical
navel bleeding: omphalorrhagia
navel center: acromphalus
navel discharge: omphalorrhea
navel excision: omphalectomy,
umbilectomy
navel hernia: liparomphalus,
omphalocele
navel incision: omphalotomy
navel inflammation: omphalitis,
omphalophlebitis
navel protrusion: acromphalus,
exomphalos, omphalocele
navel rupture: omphalorrhexis
navel-shaped: umbilicate
navel surgery: omphalotripsy
navel tumor: omphaloncus,
varicomphalus
near: juxta-, para-, peri-
nearest: proximate
nearsighted: brachymetropia, myopia
necessary: compulsive, fundamental,
obligate, vital
neck: cervic-, cervico-, trachelo-,
cervix, jugulum, nape, nucha,
throat
neck, back: dorsinuchal, nape, nucha,
retrocollic
neck, study of: trachelology
neck bruise: trachelematoma
neck diseases: retrocollis, torticollis,
trachelism
neck inflammation: trachelomyitis
neck muscles: scalene, semispinalis,
sternocleidomastoid, sternohyoid,
thyrohyoid
neck pain: cervicodynia, trachelodynia
necrosed: sphacelate
necrosed tissue: slough, sphacelus
necrosis removal: necrectomy,
necronectomy, necrotomy

needle: acu-, acus, hyperdermic, trocar
needle holder: acutenaculum
needles, fear of: belonephobia
needle-shaped: acicular, aciform,
aculeate, acuminate, belonoid,
mucronate, spicule, styloid,
umbilicate
negative: mis-
nematode diseases: dracunculiasis,
loaiasis
nematodes: Dracunculus, Loa
neoplasm: cancer, neoformation,
tumor
nerve: neur-, neuro-, afferent,
efferent, motor
See also cranial nerves
nerve, sensory: proprioceptor
nerve, toward: adnerval
nerve cavities: neurocele, neurocoele
nerve cell action: discharge
nerve cell destruction: neuronophagia
nerve cells: axon, dendraxon, dendrite,
dendron, ganglion, glia,
karyochrome, myelin sheath,
neurocyte, neurodendrite,
neuroglia, neuron, node of Ranvier,
Schwann cell, teledendrite,
telodendron
nerve chemical: acetylcholine,
catecholamine, dopamine,
neurotransmitter, norepinephrine,
serotonin
nerve conduction, absent: adromia
nerve covering: endoneurium,
epineurium
nerve crushing: neurotripsy
nerve development: neurogenesis
nerve diseases: amyotropic lateral
sclerosis, athetosis, autonomic
hyperreflexia, ballism, carpel
tunnel syndrome, cauda equina
syndrome, causalgia syndrome,
chorea, Collet-Sicard syndrome,
Creutzfeldt-Jakob disease,
demyelination, Eaton-Lambert
syndrome, entrapment syndrome,
Hallervorden-Spatz disease,
Huntington's disease,
hydranencephaly, kuru,

mononeuropathy, myasthenia
gravis, neuroarthropathy,
neurofibromatosis, neuromatosis,
neuropathy, Parkinson's,
polyneuropathy, sciatica, St. Vitus
dance, Sydenham's chorea, tarsal
tunnel syndrome, tic douloureux
nerve disease treatment: neuroleptic,
neurotherapeutics, neurotherapy
nerve displacement: neurectopia
nerve ending: baroreceptor, ceptor,
chemoreceptor, cholinergic,
exteroceptor, interoceptor,
photoreceptor, pressoreceptor,
proprioceptor, receptor, root,
tangoreceptor
nerve excision: neurectomy,
sympathectomy, sypathicectomy
nerve fibers: lemniscus, medullated,
myelinated, nonmyelinated
nerve fibers, absence: aneurogenic
nerve gap: synapse
nerve impulses, abnormal: antidromic
nerve incision: neurotomy
nerve inflammation: actinoneuritis,
Guillain-Barre syndrome, neuritis,
neurochoroiditis, neurogangliitis,
neuromyelitis, neuromyositis,
neuronitis, neurothecitis,
polyneuritis, radioneuritis, sciatica,
sympathiconeuritis
nerve inflammation preventive:
antineuritic
nerve injury: neurotmesis,
neurotrauma, neurotrosis
nerve junction: synapse
nerve malnutrition:
neurotrophasthenia
nerve-muscle spasms: neuroclonia,
neurophonia, neurospasm
nerve nutrition: neurotrophy
nerve origin: neurogenic
nerve pain: neuralgia, neurodynia,
polyneuralgia, prosopalgia,
radiculalgia, sciatica, trigeminal
neuralgia

nerve pathway: reflex arc
nerve poison: neurotoxin
nerve puncture: neuronyxis
nerve removal: denervation,
enervation
nerve repair: neurocladism,
neurotization, odogenesis
nerve root: radix
nerve root disease:
radiculomyelopathy, radiculopathy
nerve root inflammation: funiculitis,
polyradiculitis, radiculitis,
radiculomeningomyelitis,
radiculoneuritis
nerve root pain: radiculalgia
nerve root surgery: radicotomy,
radiculectomy, rhizotomy
nerves, cranial: olfactory, optic,
oculomotor, trochlear, trigeminal,
abducens, facial, vestibulocochlear,
glossopharyngeal, vagal, accessory,
hypoglossal
nerve sheath: neurilemma,
neurolemma, perineurium, sheath
of Schwann
nerve sheath inflammation:
perineuritis
nerve specialist: neurologist,
neurosurgeon
nerve stimulant: amphetamine,
analeptic
nerve stretching: neurolysis,
neurotension
nerve surgery: hersage, neuroplasty,
neurorrhaphy, neurosarcocleisis,
neurotripsy, sympathectomy,
vagotomy
nerve swelling: choked disk
nerve tissue: neuroglia
nerve tissue hardening: neurosclerosis
nerve tissue softening: neuromalacia
nerve tract incision: tractotomy
nerve tumors: glioma, neurilemoma,
neurinoma, neuroblastoma,
neurocytoma, neuroepithelioma,
neurofibroma, neurofibrosarcoma,
neuroglioma, neuroma

nervous energy: neurodynamia
nervous system: autonomic, central,
  parasympathetic, peripheral,
  sympathetic
nervous system, central: axion, brain
  and spinal cord, cerebrospinal axis
nervous system, study of:
  neuroanatomy, neurology,
  neurophysiology
nervous system stimulant:
  amphetamine, analeptic, caffeine,
  doxapram, ephedrine,
  methylphenidate, pemoline
nervous system tumors: astrocytoma,
  glioblastoma, spongioblastoma
network: plexus, rete, reticulum
network-like: plexiform, reticular,
  reticulated, retiform, textiform
neural: axonal, cerebrospinal, dendric,
  ganglial, medullary, sensory
neuralgia reliever: antineuralgic
neurocutaneous diseases: epiloia,
  tuberous sclerosis
neuroglia: amphicyte, astrocyte,
  ependyma, microglia, neurilemma,
  oligodendroglia, Schwann cell
neurologic disorder: apraxia
neuromuscular blockers: atracurium,
  gallamine, metocurine,
  pancuronium, succinylcholine,
  tubocuraine, vecuronium
neuroses: anxiety, compulsion,
  depression, fixation,
  hypochondriacal, hysteria,
  obsession, psychosocial disorder,
  somatoform disorder
neurotransmitters: catecholamine,
  dopamine, norepinephrine,
  serotonin
neuter: asexual, castrated,
  emasculated, eunuch
new: ceno-, neo-
newborn: baby, infant, neonate
newborn, study of: neonatology
newness, fear of: cainotophobia,
  centophobia, kainophobia,
  neophobia

next to: proximate
nick: blemish, bruise, scratch, wound
night: nycto-
night, fear of: noctiphobia,
  noctophobia, nyctophobia,
  scotophobia
night, love of: nyctophilia, scotophilia
night blindness: nyctalopia,
  nyctotyphlosis
nightmare: incubus, night terror,
  nocturnus, oneirodynia, paroniria,
  pavor nocturnus
nightmare preventive: antephialtic
nightshade: belladonna
nightwalking: noctambulism,
  sleepwalking, somnambulism
ninth cranial nerve: glossopharyngeal
nipple: thel-, thelo-, mamma, mamilla,
  papilla, staphylion, thelium
  See also breast
nipple, multiple: polythelia
nipple, small: microthelia
nipple area: areola
nipple bleeding: thelorrhage
nipple discharge: colostrum, milk
nipple disease: Paget's
nipple erection: thelerethism,
  thelothism
nipple inflammation: acromastititis,
  mamillitis, thelitis
nipple-like: mamillation, mamilliform,
  papilla
nipple pain: thelalgia
nipple surgery: mamilliplasty,
  theleplasty
nipple-shaped: mamilliform
nipple tumor: theloncus
nipple venous circle:
  thelophlebostemma
nitrogen: azo-
nitrogen in blood, excessive: azotemia,
  hypernitremia, uremia
nitrogen in feces, excessive: azotorrhea
nitrogen in urine, excessive: azoturia,
  hyperazoturia
nocuous: noxious, toxic, virulent

nodding: nutation
node: *See* lymph node .
nodule: apophysis, caruncle, cyst,
 mass, neoplasm, polyp, tubercle,
 tuberculum, tuberosity, tumor,
 wart, wen
nodule, small: miliary
nodules, multiple: tuberculate
noise, on hearing: socioacusis
noiseless: aphonic
noise sensitivity: oxyecoia
noncancerous: benign
nonidentical twins: dizygotic, fraternal
nonpoisonous: atoxic
nonproductive: sterile
nonpurulent: apyetous, apyogenous,
 apyous
nonpyrogenic: apyrogenic
normal: eu-, ortho-
normal, away from: deviation
normal physique: mesomorph
northern lights, fear of: auroraphobia
nose: naso-, rhin-, rhino-, naris,
 nasus, nostril, olfactory
nose, absence: anaric
nose, around: perirhinal
nose, large: macrorhinia, rhinophyma
nose, originating in: rhinogenous
nose, pointed: oxyrhine
nose, science of: rhinology
nose, slender: leptorhine
nose, small: microrhinia
nose, study of: nasology
nose, wall of: ala
nose, wide: pachyrhine
nosebleed: epistaxis, rhinorrhagia
nose bridge: dorsonasal
nose bridge depression: nasion
nose calculus: rhinodacryolith,
 rhinolith, rhinopharyngolith
nose deformity: rhinokyphosis
nose discharge: rhinorrhea
nose discharge producing: errhine
nose diseases: ozena, rhinomycosis,
 rhinonecrosis, rhinopathy,
 rhinoscleroma, rhinosporidiosis

nose dryness: xeromycteria
nose examination: rhinoscopy
nose excision: rhinocanthectomy
nose incision: rhinotomy
nose inflammation: catarrh, coryza,
 endorhinitis, nasitis, nasoantritis,
 nasopharyngitis, nasoseptitis,
 nasosinusitis, rhinitis,
 rhinoantritis, rhinopharangitis,
 rhinosalpingitis
nose mucosa: schneiderian membrane
nose obstruction: rhinocleisis,
 rhinostenosis
nose pain: rhinalgia, rhinodynia
nose plastic surgery: rhinoplasty,
 tagliacotian
nose plug: rhinobyon
nose polyps: rhinopolypus
nose specialist: rhinologist
nose surgery: rhinocheiloplasty,
 rhinomiosis, rhinommectomy
nose tumor: rhinopharyngocele
nostrum: patent medicine
not: a-, an-, non-, un-
not paired: azygous
notch: crenate, dentate, fold, furrow,
 incision, incisura, ridge, serrate
nourishment: nutri-, trop-, troph-,
 -trophy, alimentation,
 hyperalimentation, nutriment
novelty, fear of: cainotophobia,
 cenotophobia
noxious: foul, lethal, mephitic,
 pernicious, poisonous, toxic,
 virulent
nucleus: cary-, caryo-, karyo-, nucle-,
 nucleo-, cytoblast, karyon,
 karyoplast
nucleus, chromatin network:
 karyomitome
nucleus, division: karyokinesis
nucleus, fibrillar network:
 karyoreticulum, linin
nucleus, liquid matter: karyolymph
nucleus, lobe-shaped: karyolobic
nucleus, multiple: polykaryocyte,
 polynuclear

nucleus, resting stage: karyostasis
nucleus, shape: karyomorphism,
    karyospherical
nucleus, stainable: karyochromatophil
nucleus, study of: karyology
nucleus, within: karyozoic
nucleus, without: denucleated,
    enucleated
nucleus break down: karyoklasis
nucleus destruction: karyolysis,
    karyorrhexis, necrobiosis
nucleus division: prophase, metaphase,
    anaphase, telaphase, interphase;
    meiosis, mitosis
nucleus enlargement, abnormal:
    karyomegaly
nucleus formation: karyogenesis
nucleus fusion: synkaryon
nucleus-like: nucleiform, nucleoid
nucleus measurement: karyometry
nucleus membrane: karyotheca
nucleus phagocyte: karyophage
nucleus protoplasm: karyoplasm,
    nucleoplasm
nucleus rupture: karyorrhexis
nucleus skrinkage: karyopyknosis
numbness: narco-, anesthesize,
    hemiparesthesia, hypnosis,
    narcohypnia, narcosis, obdormition,
    paralysis, paresthesia, shock, topor
nurse: breastfeed, suckle, treat
nursemaid's elbow: radial subluxation
nursing: nosotrophy
nursing behavior: assessing,
    analyzing, planning,
    implementing, evaluation
nutrition: -trophy
nutrition disorder: trophopathy,
    trophotonos, vitamin deficiency
nutrition, science of: sitiology,
    sitology, trophology
nutritive: alible
nystagmus-like: nystagmoi

O

obesity: adipose, corpulence,
    pickwickian syndrome
    See also fat
obesity, science of: bariatrics
obey: compliance
obituary: necrology
object manipulation, impaired: apraxia
oblivious: amnesic
oblong: thyreo-, thyro-, ovoid
obscure: obfuscation, occult
obsession: complex, compulsion,
    delusion, fixation, hallucination,
    idee fixe, illusion, impulse, mania,
    nookleptia, nympholepsy, phobia
obsessive-compulsive: anancastia
obstetrician: accoucheur
obstetrics: tocology
obstruct: occlude, occlusion
obstruction: blockage, constipation,
    emphraxis, ileus, obstruent,
    obturation, occlusion, oppilation,
    stegnosis, stenosis
occasional: intermittent, periodic
occlusion: -atresia, synizesis
occult: hidden, obscure
occupational diseases: acro-osteolysis,
    aluminosis, anthracosilicosis,
    anthracosis, asbestosis, asthma,
    bagassosis, berylliosis, birth
    defects, bituminosis, byssinosis,
    cadmiosis, cannabosis,
    cardiotoxicity, chalicosis, cyanide
    poisoning, decarborane poisoning,
    dermatitis, diborane poisoning,
    green tobacco sickness, kaolinosis,
    leukemia, nystagmus, pentaborane
    poisoning, pneumoconiosis,
    sarcoidosis, siderosis, silicosis,
    sterility, stress
occurrence frequency: incidence,
    prevalence
occurring continuously: endemic
ocular: ophthalmic, optical
    See also eye, vision

oculist: ophthalmologist, optometrist
odd: aberrant, abnormal, amorphous, anomalous, atypical, deviant, teratological
odor: brom-, bromo-, osmo-, osphresio-, effluvium, emanation, osmyl
See also smell
odor, bad: bromidrosis, cacosmia, fetor, mephitic, ozocrotia
odor, dislike of: osmodysphoria
odor, fear of: bromidrosiphobia, olfactophobia, osmophobia, osphresiophobia
odor, love of: osphresiophilia
odor, science of: osmology, osphresiology
odor sensitivity: hyperosmia, osmesthesia
off: ab-, abs-
offensive: aggressive, mephitic, nauseating, putrescent, putrid
offset: antidote, buffer, juxtapose, neurtralize
offspring: child, clone, descendant, fetus, infant, neonate, progeny
oil: eleo-, oleo-, balm, liniment, lubricant, ointment, olein, oleum, petrolatum, petroleum, pomatum, salve, triolein, unguent
oil treatment: oleoarthrosis, oleotherapy, oleothorax
oily: oleaginous, oleoresinous, oleosus, sebaceous, unctuous
ointment: abirritant, balm, cerate, demulcent, embrocation, liniment, lubricant, magma, palliative, salve, unction, unguent
old: paleo-
old age: gero-, geronto-, presby-, anility, dotage, senescence, senilism, senility
old age, study of: gereology, geriatrics, gerontology, presbyatrics
olecranon-like: olecranoid

omentum: epiploon
omentum inflammation: epiploitis, omentitis
omentum surgery: epiplopexy, omentectomy, omentopexy, omentorrhaphy, omentosplenopexy, omentotomy
on: em-, en-, ep-, epi-
one: mon-, mono-, uni-, azygos, individual
one-armed: monobrachius
one-eyed: cyclopia, monocular, monophthalia, uniocular
oneness: compatibility
oneself: idio-, ego
one-sided: asymmetric
ongoing: chronic, habitual, recurrent
onset: genesis
ooze: discharge, drain, exudation, flow, perspiration, secretion, sweat, transudation
opalescent: mottling, polychromatic
opaque: turbid
open: dehiscent, distended, patent, patulous, perforate
open fracture: compound fracture
opening: ampulla, aperture, areola, cardia, cavity, channel, crevice, fenestra, fissure, foramen, hiatus, interstice, introitus, lacuna, meatus, orifice, os, osculum, ostium, ostomy, pore, porta, punctum, pupil, sinus, slit, stoma, vent, window
opening, abnormal: fistula
opening, absence: atreto-, atresia, imperforate, occluded
opening, artificial: ostomy
See also specific organs
opening, blocked: atresia, clausura, obturator.
opening in abdomen: colostomy, cyolostomy, enterostomy, ileostomy, ostomy
openings, multiple: polystomatous
open spaces, fear of: agoraphobia, claustrophilia

open spaces, love of: agoraphilia
operation: *See* specific organ, surgery
opiates: analgesic, endorphin,
enkephalin, hypnotic, narcotic,
sedative, somnifacient, soporific,
stupefacient
opium: codeine, heroin, laudanum,
morphine, papaverine, paregoric
opium addiction: narcotism,
opiophagism, opiumism
opposing action: antagonist
opposite: anti-, contra-, antipodal
opposite side: contralateral, contrecoup
optic: ocular, ophthalmic
See also eye, vision
optic disk inflammation: papillitis
optic disk swelling: choked disk,
papilledema
optic nerve disease: neuroretinopathy
optic nerve inflammation:
neuroretinitis, postocular neuritis,
retrobulbar neuritis
optimistic: sanguine
oral: os, verbal
oral herpes: herpes simplex
oral intercourse: fellatio
orb: eyeball, orbit, spherical
organ: parenchyma, stroma
See also tissue
organ, abnormal: dysgenesis
organ, absence: agenesis, aplasia
organ development: organogenesis,
organogeny
organ displacement: splanchnectopia
organic: animate, biotic, innate
organlike: organoid
organs, internal: splanchnic, visceral
organs, study of: anatomy,
organology, physiology
orgasm, lack of: anorgasmia
oriental sore: cutaneous leishmaniasis
orientation: adaptation, assimilation,
placement
orifice: pyle-, aperture, areola, cavity,
fenestra, foramen, interstice,
lacuna, mouth, ostium, perforation,
puncture, sinus, stoma

origin: embryo, etiology, genesis,
germination, primordium
origin, multiple: polyphyletic
origin, one: monophyletic
origin, within: endogenous
origin, without: exogenous
original: arch-, arche-, archi-,
archetype, precursor, primordial,
princeps, prototype
original condition: primary
original subject: index case, proband,
propositus
origin unknown: agnogenic,
cryptogenic, idiopathic
ornithosis: Chlamydia, psittacosis
orthopedic devices: brace, splint,
traction
orthoses: airplane splint, Balkan
frame, body jacket, Bradford
frame, Bryant's traction, Buck's
traction, Kydex body jacket, Lenox
Hill brace, Milwaukee brace,
Philadelphia collar, spica cast,
Taylor-Knight, Thomas splint,
traction splint, truss, turnbuckle
cast
oscillating: pendulous
oscillations: fluctuations, vibrations
other: allo-, heter-, hetero-
outbreak: epidemic, eruption,
manifestation
outburst: convulsion, paroxysm,
seizure, spasm, tantrum
outcome: sequela
outer part: cortic-, cortico-, cortex,
integument, skin
outflow: discharge, effluvium, effusion,
ejaculation
outgrowth: ecphyma, excrescence,
exophytic, exostosis, node, nodule,
poroma, process, protuberance
outlet: aperture, artery, channel,
drain, duct, emissary, passage,
vessel
out of: ec-
outpouring: effluvium, effusion

outside: ecto-, ex-, exo-, extra-,
external, extrinsic, peripheral
outward: exo-, efferent, extroversion
oval: oviform, ovoid
ovary: oari-, oario-, ooario-, oopho-,
oophor-, oophoro-, ovari-, ovario-,
corpus albicans, corpus luteum,
graafian follicle, oophoron, ootheca,
ovarium, ovum
ovary, abnormal: hyperovaria,
hypovaria, oopharauxe
ovary, absence: agenosomia,
anovarism
ovary, pregnancy in: ovariocyesis
ovary abscess: pyoovarium
ovary bleeding: oophorrhagia
ovary cyst: hydrovarium
ovary cyst formation: oophorocystosis
ovary diseases: oophoropathy,
ovariopathy
ovary excision: castration,
gonadectomy, oophorectomy,
oophorocystectomy,
oophorohysterectomy,
oophorosalpingectomy,
oothecohysterectomy, ovariectomy,
ovariohysterectomy,
ovariosalpingectomy, ovariosteresis,
ovarnectomy, salpingo-
oophorecotomy, tuboovariotomy
ovary fixation: adnexopexy,
oophoropexy, ovariopexy
ovary hernia: ovariocele
ovary incision: ovariotomy
ovary inflammation: oophoritis,
oophorosalpingitis,
ovariosalpingitis, ovaritis,
perioophoritis,
perioophorosalpingitis,
perioothecitis,
perioothecosalpingitis,
perisalpingoovaritis,
perisalpingitis, pyosalpingo-
oophoritis, sclero-oophoritis
ovary malfunction: anovulation
ovary pain: mittelschmerz,
oophoralgia, ovarialgia,
ovariodysneuria

ovary puncture: ovariocentesis
ovary rupture: ovariorrhexis
ovary surgery: oophoroplasty,
oophorostomy, ovariostomy
ovary suturing: oophorrhaphy
ovary tumors: andreoblastoma,
arrhenoblastoma, gyroma,
masculinovoblastoma, oophoroma,
thecoma
over: supra-, trans-
overbite: malocclusion
overcrowding, disease from: ochlesis
overfeeding: hypernutrition
overgrowth: giga-, gigantism,
hyperplasia, hypertrophy,
superinfection
overhang: permeate, pervade
overlap: imbricate
overripe: hypermature
oversized: macr-, macro-
overt: conscious, patent
over-the-counter: nonprescription
overweight: fat, obesity
overwrought: hysterical
oviduct: fallopian tube
oviduct twisting: syringosystrophy,
tubotorsion
ovum: oo-, ovi-, ovo-, gamete, oocyte,
ootid
ovum, absence: anovulation
ovum, fertilized: arsenoblast, cytula,
oosperm, pronucleus, spermatovum,
zygocyte, zygote
ovum production: oogenesis,
oviogenesis
oxalates in urine, excessive:
hyperoxaluria, oxalosis
oxygen: oxy-
oxygen, life in: aerobic
oxygen, life without: anaerobic,
anaerobiosis
oxygen deficiency: anoxia, asphyxia,
hypoxemia, hypoxia, mionectic,
supervenosity
oxygen saturation: pleonectic
oyster poisoning: ostreotoxism

P

pace: gait
pacer: pacemaker
pacify: abate, alleviate, palliate,
   relieve, tranquilize
pack: agglomerate, compact,
   compress, conglobate,
   conglomerate, constrict, tampon,
   tamponade
pad: bandage, compress, dressing,
   fascia, gauze, pledget
pain: -agra, alg-, alge-, algesi-,
   -algia, algo-, -odynia, odyno-,
   ache, algos, dolor, dyspraxia, labor,
   paralgesia, paralgia, stitch, throb,
   twinge
pain, absence: analgesia, analgia,
   anodynia, apronia
pain, burning: causalgia, thermalgia
pain, fear of: algophobia, odynophobia
pain, generalized: pantalgia
pain, hysterical: algopsychalia,
   phrenalgia, psychalgia
pain, localized: topoalgia
pain, love of: algophily, masochism
pain, menstrual: algomenorrhea,
   dysmenorrhea
pain, referred: synalgia,
   synesthesialgia, telalgia
pain, related to: -algic
pain, sensitiveness to: algesia,
   algesthesia
pain, severe: megalgia
pain, study of: algology, dolorology
pain-free: analgia, anesthetized
pain from heat: thermalgia,
   thermohyperalgia
pain from light: photalgia, photodynia
painful: dys-, algesic, algetic
painful intercourse: dyspareunia,
   dyspermia
painful urination: alginuresis, dysuria,
   urodynia
pain in abdomen: abdominalgia,
   celiomyalgia, splanchnodynia

pain in anesthetized area: analgesia
   algera, anesthesia dolorosa
pain in ankle: talalgia
pain in aorta: aortalgia
pain in appendix: appendalgia
pain in arm: brachialgia
pain in artery: arterialgia
pain in back: dorsalgia, dorsodynia,
   lumbago, lumbodynia, notalgia,
   rachialgia
pain in bile ducts: cholecystalgia
pain in bones: ostealgia, osteocope,
   osteodynia, osteoneuralgia
pain in breast: mammalgia, mastalgia,
   mastodynia
pain in buttocks: pygalgia
pain in carotid artery: carotidynia,
   carotodynia
pain in chest: acute myocardial
   infarction, angina, cardialgia,
   cardiodynia, dissecting aortic
   aneurysm, hiatus hernia,
   hyperventilation, pectoralgia,
   pericarditis, pleuralgia,
   pleurodynia, pneumothorax,
   precordialgia, pulmonary embolus,
   thoracalgia, thoracodynia
pain in colon: colalgia, colonalgia
pain in cornea: keratalgia
pain in cricoid cartilage: cricoidynia
pain in diaphragm: diaphragmalgia,
   diaphragmodynia, phrenalgia,
   phrenodynia
pain in dreams: hypnalgia
pain in ear: odynacusis, otalgia,
   otodynia, otoneuralgia
pain in elbow: epicondylalgia
pain in esophagus: esophagalgia
pain in extremities: acroesthesia,
   brachialgia, melagra, melalgia
pain in eye: heterophoralgia,
   ophthalmagra, ophthalmalgia,
   ophthalmodynia, photalgia
pain in face: erythroprosopalgia,
   opsialgia
pain in foot: metatarsalgia, pedialgia,
   pedionalgia, podalgia, pododynia,
   tarsalgia

pain in gallbladder: cholecystalgia
pain in glands: adenalgia, adenodynia
pain in groin: inguinodynia
pain in gums: gingivalgia
pain in half of body: hemialgia
pain in hand and arm: graphospasm
pain in head: cephalalgia,
  cephalodynia, clavus,
  encephalalgia, headache,
  hemicrania, migraine
pain in heel: calcaneodynia,
  calcanodynia, talalgia
pain in hip: coxalgia, coxodynia,
  ischialgia, ischioneuralgia, sciatica
pain in iris: iridalgia
pain in jaw: gnathalgia, gnathodynia
pain in joint: arthralgia, arthrodynia,
  arthroneuralgia
pain in kidney: nephralgia,
  nephrocolic
pain in knee: gonalgia
pain in labor: parodynia
pain in lacrimal glands:
  dacryadenalgia, dacrycystalgia,
  dacryoadenalgia
pain in ligament: desmalgia,
  desmodynia
pain in lip: cheilalgia
pain in liver: hepatalgia, hepatodynia
pain in mastoid: mastoidalgia
pain in mouth: stomatalgia,
  stomatodynia
pain in muscle: kinesalgia, kinesialgia,
  myalgia, myocelialgia, myodynia,
  myosalgia, pleurodynia
pain in nails: onychalgia
pain in neck: cervicodynia
pain in nerve: neuralgia, neurodynia,
  polyneuralgia, radiculalgia, sciatica
pain in nipple: thelalgia
pain in ovary: mittelschmerz,
  oophoralgia, ovarialgia,
  ovariodysneuria
pain in pancreas: pancreatalgia
pain in penis: phallalgia, phallodynia,
  priapism

pain in pharynx: pharayngalgia,
  pharyngodynia
pain in pleura: parapleuritis,
  pleuralgia, pleurodynia
pain in rectum: proctagra, proctalgia,
  proctodynia, rectalgia
pain in retina: neurodealgia
pain in rib: costalgia, pleurodynia
pain in sacroiliac joint: sacrocoxalgia
pain in sacrum: hieralgia, sacralgia,
  sacrodynia
pain in shoulder: omalgia, omodynia,
  scapulalgia, scapulodynia
pain in sinus: genyantralgia
pain in skin: dermalgia, dermatalgia,
  dermatodynia, erythralgia
pain in spermatic cord:
  spermoneuralgia
pain in sphincter ani: sphincteralgia
pain in spinal cord: myealgia
pain in spine: rachialgia, rachiodynia
pain in spleen: spinalgia, splenalgia,
  splenodynia
pain in sternum: sternalgia,
  sternodynia
pain in stomach: cardialgia,
  gastralgia, gastrodynia,
  peratodynia, stomachalgia
pain in subcostal nerve: subcostalgia
pain in sympathetic ganglion:
  sympatheticalgia
pain in tendons: tenalgia, tenodynia,
  tenontodynia
pain in testes: didymalgia, orchialgia,
  orchidalgia, orchiodynia,
  orchioneuralgia
pain in thigh: meralgia
pain in thigh and hip: merocoxalgia
pain in tibia: tibialgia
pain in tongue: glossalgia, glossodynia
pain in tooth: aerodontalgia,
  dentalgia, odontagra, odontalgia,
  odontia, odontodynia
pain in trachea: trachealgia
pain in ureter: ureteralgia
pain in urethra: spondylalgia,
  urethralgia

pain in uterus: hysteralgia,
hysterodynia, metralgia,
metrodynia, uteralgia
pain in vagina: colpalgia
pain in vessels: vasalgia
pain in xiphoid process: xiphodynia
painkiller: acesodyne, acetylsalicylic
acid, acupressure, analgesic,
analgesic cocktail, andioanesthesia,
anesthetic, anodyne, antalgesic,
barbiturate, desensitization, drug,
electroanalgesia, endorphins,
enkephalins, hypnotic, lytic
cocktail, morphine, narcotic, opiate,
sedative, soporific
painlessness, partial: hemianalgesia,
hemianesthesia
pain measurement: algesichronometer,
algesiometer, odynometry
pain on swallowing: odynophagia
pain perception: nociperception
pain producing: algesiogenic,
algogenic, dolorific, dolorogenic
pain relief, study of: anesthesiology
pain sensation, absence of: analgesia
pain sensitivity: algesia, algesthesia,
hyperesthesia
pain sensitivity, increased:
hyperalgesia, hyperalgia,
hyperpathia
pain sensitivity, reduced: hypalgia,
hypalgesia
pain sensitivity measurement:
algesiometry, ponography
pain spasm: throe
pain therapy: acupuncture,
biofeedback, massage, moxibustion,
pharmaceuticals, relaxation
pain transmitter: nociceptor
pair: bi-, diplo-, zygo-, binary, dyad,
twins
paired: bigeminal, conjugate
palate: palato-, urano-, palatum,
uraniscus, velum
palate, cleft: palatognathous,
palatoschisis, staphylochisis,
uraniscochasma

palate, hard: palatum durum
palate, paralyzed: palatoplegia
palate, soft: palatum molle, velum
palatinum
palate inflammation: palatitis,
uranisconitis
palate mass: cion, staphyle, uvula
palate movement recording:
palatography
palate paralysis, soft: palatoplegia,
uranoplegia
palate surgery: platoplasty,
palatorrhaphy, staphyloplasty,
staphylorrhaphy, uranoplasty
palate suturing: palatorrhaphy
pale: achromatic, anemic, etiolation,
pallescence, pallid, pallor
palliative: abirritant, analgesic,
anesthetic, demulcent, emollient,
lenitive, narcotic, opiate, sedative,
tranquilizer, unguent
palm: thenar, volar, manus,
antethenar, hypothenar eminence,
thenar eminence
palm, face downward: pronation
palm, face upward: supination
palm, toward: thenad
palm prominence: antithenar,
hypothenar eminence, thenar
eminence
palpation: examination, manipulation,
massage, stereognosis
palpitation: ballottement, palmus,
pulsation, tremor, trepidation,
vibration
palsy: Bell's, cerebral, Erb's, paralysis,
Parkinson's disease, paralysis
agitans
pancreas: islets of Langerhans
pancreas, decreased secretion:
hypopancreatism
pancreas, excessive secretion:
hyperpancreatism
pancreas, normal: eupancreatism
pancreas, produced by:
pancreatogenic

pancreas calculus: pancreatolith, pancreatolithiasis
pancreas destruction: pancreatolysis
pancreas diseases: dyspancreatism, dystrypsia, pancreathelcosis, pancreatopathy, pancreopathy
pancreas excision: depancreatize, pancreatectomy, pancreatoduodenectomy, pancreatothectomy, pancreectomy
pancreas incision: pancreatomy, pancreatotomy
pancreas inflammation: pancreatitis, peripancreatitis
pancreas pain: pancreatalgia
pancreas surgery: pancreaticocholecystostomy, pancreaticoduodenostomy, pancreaticoenterostomy, pancreaticogastrostomy, pancreaticojejunostomy, pancreatolithotomy, pancreolithotomy
pancreas swelling: pancreatemphraxis
pancreas tumor: gastrinoma, glucagonoma, pancreatoncus
pandemic: epidemic, pestilence, plague, zymosis
pang: ache, pain, spasm
pant: dyspnea, hyperventilate, hyperpnea, polypnea
papilla excision: papillectomy
papule: caruncle, comedo, milium, papilla, pustule
paraffin hydrocarbons: -ane
paralysis: -plegia, anesthetized, bulbar, palsy, paresis, polyparesis, polyplegia, pseudobulbar, stroke
paralysis, lack of: aparalytic
paralysis, partial: diplegia, hemiparesis, hemiplegia, monoplegia, paraplegia, poliomyelitis, semisideratio, triplegia
paralysis, relief of: antiparalytic
paralysis of arms: Erb's palsy

paralysis of extremities: paraplegia, quadriplegia, tetraplegia
paranasal sinus inflammation: pansinusitis
parasite: cestode, entozoon, paratrophic
parasite, fear of: parasitophobia
parasite, study of: parasitology
parasite disease: *See* blood flukes, flukes, worms
parasite therapy: *See* anthelmintics
parathyroid, decreased activity: hypoparathyroidism
parathyroid, overactivity: hyperparathyroidism
parathyroid disease: parathyroprivia
parathyroid excision: parathyroidectomy
parched: anhydrous, dehydrated, desiccated, evaporated, exsiccated
parenchyma inflammation: parenchymatitis
parent: progenitor
parentage: heredity, pedigree
parkinsonian therapy: antiparkinsonian
parotid gland inflammation: parotitis
paroxysm: convulsion, eclampsia, epilepsy, ictus, jactitation, seizure, spasm, tantrum, tetanus, throe, tremor
parrot fever: Chlamydia, ornithosis, psittacosis
part: mero-, abarticulation, bifurcation, cleft, disjunction, fissure, limb, membrane, organ, pars, partio, structure, tissue
particle: atom, granule, molecule
particles, localized: anachoresis
particularize: differentiate
partition: diaphragm, dissepiment, mediastinum, membrane, septulum, septum, wall
parturition: accouchement, eutocia
  See also childbirth, delivery, labor
pass: defecate, discharge, egestion, eliminate, evacuate, excrete, expel, micturate, urinate, void

passage: aperture, aqueduct, canal,
    canaliculus, channel, duct, fiber,
    fistula, foramen, lumen, orifice,
    tube
passage formation: canalization,
    fistulization
passion, sexual: aphrodisia
passive: dormant, vegetative
pass urine: micturate, urinate, void
paste: cataplasm, magma, mucilage,
    poultice
pasty: anemic, mucilaginous, pallid,
    visid
patches: areata
patella-like: patelliform
patent medicine: nostrum
pathology: anatomopathology,
    diagnostics, etiology,
    nosochthonography, nosogenesis,
    nosology, pathogenesis,
    pathognomy
pathway: channel, course, duct, fiber,
    tract
patient: convalescent, valetudinarian
pattern: model, prototype, template
paunch: abdomen
peak: apex, crown, vertex
peaked: anemic, emaciated, pallid
pearly: iridescent, opalescent, opaque
pear-shaped: piriform
pea-shaped: pisiform
pectoral: respiratory, thoracic, ventral
peculiarity: aberration, anomaly,
    characteristic, deviation, trait
pedigree: heredity
peel: desquamate, excoriate, shed,
    slough
peeping Tom: voyeur
peg-leg: pillion, pylon
pelvis: pyelo-, coccyx bones,
    innominate, sacrum
pelvis, broad: platypellic
pelvis, long: dolichopellic
pelvis, narrow: leptopellic
pelvis examination: pelvioscopy
pelvis inflammation: pelvioperitonitis

pelvis surgery: pelvioplasty,
    pelviotomy, pubiotomy,
    symphysiotomy
penetration: impregnation, incision,
    infusion, perforation, puncture,
    saturation, transfusion
penicillins: amdiocillin, amoxicillin,
    ampicillin, azlocillin, bacampicillin,
    carbenicillin, clavulanic acid,
    cloxacillin, cyclocillin, didoxacillin,
    hetacillin, methicillin, mezlocillin,
    nafcillin, oxacillin, penicillin G,
    penicillin V, piperacillin, ticarcillin
penis: phallo-, glans, membrum virile,
    phallus, prepuce, preputium,
    smegma, tentum
penis, artificial: dildo
penis, double: diphallus
penis, glans: balano-
penis, large: macrophallus,
    megalopenis, mentulate
penis, small: microcaulia, microphallus
penis bleeding: phallarhagia
penis discharge: ejaculate, semen,
    seminal fluid, sperm, urine
penis diseases: anaspadias,
    balanorrhea, belanorrhagia,
    chordee, epispadias, hypspodia,
    mentulagra, paraphimosis,
    paraspadias, penischisis,
    peotillomania, Peyronie's disease,
    phallanastrophe, phallaneurysm,
    phallocampsis, phallocrypsis,
    phimosis, priapism
penis excision: phallectomy, peotomy
penis incision: phallotomy
penis inflammation: acroposthitis,
    balanitis, balanoblennorrhea,
    balanoposthitis, cavernitis,
    cavernositis, penitis, phallitis,
    posthitis, priapitis
penislike: dildo, godemiche, olisbos,
    phalliform, phalloid
penis pain: phallalgia, phallodynia,
    priapism
penis surgery: balanoplasty,
    circumcision, phalloplasty

penis tumor: phalloncus
people, fear of: anthropophobia
pepsin, absence: anapepsia
perception: -aesthesia, -esthesia,
    cognition
perception, false: allopsychosis,
    esthesia, hallucination, illusion
perception, loss of: agnosia
perception, slowness: bradyesthesia
percussion: acouophonia, plessesthesia
percussion sound: box-note, vesicular
    resonance
perforated: carious, cribrated,
    perforans, pierce, tresis
pericardium inflammation:
    pericardiomediastinitis,
    pericarditis, trichocardia
pericardium surgery:
    pericardicentesis, pericardiectomy,
    pericardiorrhaphy, pericardiopexy,
    pericardiostomy, pericardiotomy
perichondrum inflammation:
    perichondritis
perineal hernia: perineocele
perineal incision: perineotomy
perineal surgery: perineoplasty,
    perineorrhaphy
perineal suturing: episiorrhaphy
period: menstruation
period, stopping of: amenorrhea,
    menopause
periodic breathing: Cheyne-Stokes
    respiration
periodontium disease: periodontoclasis
periostium edema: periosteoedema
periostium inflammation: periosteitis,
    periostitis
periostium surgery: periosteorrhaphy,
    periosteotomy
periostium tumor: periosteoma,
    periostoma
peripheral: acentric
peristalsis: enterocinesia
peristalsis, absent: aperistalsis
peristalsis inhibitor: antiperistaltic
peristalsis reversed: anastalsis

peritoneum, fluid in: ascites,
    hydroperitoneum, seroperitoneum
peritoneum, fluid removal:
    venoperitoneostomy
peritoneum inflammation:
    ectoperitonitis, endoperitonitis,
    peritonitis, pneumoperitonitis
permeable: osmosis, porous
pernicious: fatal, lethal, malignant
persistent: chronic
person, limb missing: amputee
personality: character, ego, psyche
personality disorders: automatism,
    dissociation, dual, extrovert, fugue,
    hebephrenia, introvert, multiple,
    schizophrenia, vigilambulism
perspiration: hidro-, diaphoresis,
    hidropoiesis, sudoresis
    See also sweat
pertaining to: -alis
pervade: infiltrate, osmosis, penetrate,
    permeate, transfusion
pervert: masochist, necrophiliac,
    nymphomaniac, paraphiliac,
    pedophiliac, sadist, sodomist
pessimism: depression, melancholia
pestilence: endemic, epidemic, plague
phagocyte destruction: phagocytolysis,
    phagolysis
phagocytosis facilitation:
    opsonification, opsonization
phalanges: See digit, finger, toe
pharynx: pharyngo-
pharynx, science of: pharyngology
pharynx bleeding: pharangorrhagia
pharynx diseases: pharyngokeratosis,
    pharyngolith, pharyngolysis,
    pharyngomycosis,
    pharyngoparalysis,
    pharyngopathy, pharyngoperistole,
    pharyngoplegia, pharyngorrhea
pharynx dryness: pharyngoxerosis
pharynx examination:
    pharyngorhinoscopy,
    pharyngoscopy
pharynx hernia: pharyngocele

pharynx inflammation: halzoun,
 juxtangina, pharyngitis,
 pharyngoamygdalitis,
 pharyngolaryngitis,
 pharyngorhinitis,
 pharyngosalpingitis,
 pharyngotonsillitis
pharynx obstruction:
 pharyngemphraxis,
 pharyngostenosis
pharynx pain: pharyngalgia,
 pharyngodynia
pharynx spasm: pharyngismus,
 pharyngospasm
pharynx surgery: pharyngectomy,
 pharyngoplasty, pharyngostomy,
 pharyngotomy
pharynx treatment: pharyngotherapy
pheresis: apheresis, cytapheresis,
 erythrocytapheresis,
 erythropheresis, leukapheresis,
 lymphapheresis,
 lymphoplasmapheresis,
 plasmapheresis,
 thrombocytapheresis
phlegm: humor, mucus
phlegmatic: apathetic, lethargic
phobias: acarophobia, acerophobia,
 achluophobia, acousticophobia,
 acrophobia, aerophobia,
 agoraphobia, agrypniophobia,
 agytiophobia, aichmophobia,
 ailurophobia, algophobia,
 amathophobia, amaxophobia,
 amychophobia, androphobia,
 anemophobia, anginophobia,
 anthropophobia, antlophobia,
 apeirophobia, apiphobia,
 arachneophobia, asthenophobia,
 astraphobia, atephobia,
 auroarphobia, automyosophobia,
 autophobia, bacillophobia,
 ballistophobia, barophobia,
 basiphobia, bathophobia,
 batophobia, batrachophobia,
 belonephobia, bromidrosiphobia,
 brontophobia, categelophobia,
 cenophobia, cheimaphobia,

chionophobia, chromatophobia,
 chromophobia, chronophobia,
 cibophobia, claustrophobia,
 cleithrophobia, climacophobia,
 clithrophobia, coitophobia,
 cometophobia, coprophobia,
 cremnophobia, crystallophobia,
 cynophobia, cypridophobia,
 cypriphobia, demonomania,
 demonophobia, demophobia,
 dermatophobia, dermatosiophobia,
 dextrophobia, dikephobia,
 domatophobia, doraphobia,
 dromophobia, dysmorphophobia,
 eisoptrophobia, electrophobia,
 emetophobia, entheomania,
 entomophobia, eremophobia,
 ereuthophobia, ergasiophobia,
 ergophobia, erotophobia,
 erythrophobia, esophobia,
 eurotophobia, fibriphobia,
 galeophobia, gamophobia,
 gatophobia, genophobia,
 gephyrophobia, geumaphobia,
 graphophobia, gymnophobia,
 gynecophobia, gynophobia,
 hadephobia, hamartophobia,
 haphephobia, haptephobia,
 harpaxophobia, hedonophobia,
 heliophobia, helminthophobia,
 hematophobia, hemophobia,
 hierophobia, hodophobia,
 homichlophobia, homilophobia,
 hormephobia, hydrophobia,
 hydrophobophobia, hyelophobia,
 hygrophobia, hylophobia,
 hypengyophobia,
 hypertrichophobia, hyposophobia,
 ichthyophobia, ideophobia,
 iophobia, kainophobia,
 kainotophobia,
 kakorrhaphiophobia,
 katagelophobia, kathisophobia,
 kenophobia, keraunophobia,
 kinesophobia, kleptophobia,
 kopophobia, laliophobia, levophobia,
 linonophobia, lyssophobia,
 maieusiophobia, maniaphobia,

mechanophobia, megalophobia,
melipmophobia, melissophobia,
meningitophobia, merinthophobia,
metallophobia, meterorophobia,
microbiophobia, microphobia,
molysmophobia, monopathophobia,
monophobia, musophobia,
mysophobia, mythophobia,
necrophobia, negrophobia,
neophobia, noctiphobia, nosophobia,
nudophobia, nyctophobia,
ochlophobia, odontophobia,
odynophobia, oikophobia,
olfactophobia, ombrophobia,
ommatophobia, onomatophobia,
ophidiophobia, ornithophobia,
osmophobia, osphresiophobia,
pagonophobia, panophobia,
panphobia, pantophobia,
parasitophobia, parthenophobia,
pathophobia, patroiophobia,
peccatiphobia, pediculophobia,
pediophobia, peniaphobia,
phagophobia, pharmacophobia,
phasmophobia, phengophobia,
phobophobia, phonophobia,
photaugiophobia, photophobia,
phronemophobia, phthiriophobia,
phthisiophobia, pnigerophobia,
pnigophobia, poinephobia,
polyphobia, ponophobia,
potamophobia, proctophobia,
proteinophobia, psychophobia,
psychrophobia, pteronophobia,
pyrexeophobia, pyrophobia,
rectophobia, rhabdophobia,
rhypophobia, rupophobia,
satanophobia, scabiophobia,
sclerophobia, scopophobia,
scotophobia, siderodromophobia,
siderophobia, sitophobia,
spectrophobia, spermatophobia,
stasibasiphobia, stasiphobia,
stygiophobia, symbolophobia,
syphilophobia, tabophobia,
tachophobia, taeniphobia,
taphephobia, teratophobia,
thaassophobia, thalassophobia,
thanatophobia, theophobia,
thermophobia, topophobia,
toxicophobia, traumatophobia,
tremophobia, trichophobia,
trichopathophobia,
triskaidekophobia, tuberculophobia,
vaccinophobia, xenophobia,
zelophobia, zoophobia
phoresis: cataphoresis, electrophoresis,
immunophoresis, ionophoresis
phosphate precipitation:
phosphatoptosis
phosphates in blood, excessive:
hyperphosphatemia,
hyperphospheremia, phosphatemia
phosphates in blood, reduced:
hypophosphatemia
phosphates in urine, excessive:
hyperphosphaturia, phosphaturia,
phosphoruria, phosphuria
phosphates, reduced in urine:
hypophosphaturia,
oligophosphaturia
phosphorus deficiency: phosphopenia
phosphorus poisoning: phosphorism
physic: aperient, aperitive,
carminative, cathartic, drug,
hydragogue, laxative, medication,
medicine, pharmaceutical,
purgative
physician: iatro-, surgeon
physician caused: iatrogenic
physiologic: autoregulation,
equlibrium
pia mater inflammation:
leptomeningitis, piarachnitis, piitis
pick at bedclothes: floccillation
piebald: leukoderma, vitiligo
pierce: penetrate, perforate, puncture
pigeon breast: pectus carinatum
pigeon toed: pes varus, talipes varus
pigment: chrom-, -chromia,
adrenochrome, anthocyanin,
bilicyanin, biliflavin, bilifuscin,
biliprasin, bilipurpurin, bilrubin,
biliverdin, carotene, ceroid,
chalcone, chlorophane, chlorophyll,
choletelin, choleverdin,
cholochrome, erythropsin, fuscin,

hematin, hemin, hemofuscin,
hemoglobin, hemosiderin,
lipochrome, melanin, melanoid,
methemoglobin, myoglobin,
myohemoglobin, phymatorhusin,
pigmentum, porphyrin, purpurin,
pyoxanthine, pyoxanthose,
retinene, rhodopsin, stercobilin,
urobilin, urobilinogen, urochrome,
uroerythrin, urofuscin,
urofuscohematin, urohematin,
urolutein, uromelanin,
uroporphyrin, urorosein,
urorrhodin, urorubin,
urorubrohematin, urosacin,
urospectrin, uroxanthin,
verdohemoglobin, xanthopsis

pigment, absence: albinism,
amelanotic, leukasmus, leukoderma,
vitiligo

pigment, excessive: hyperchromatism,
hyperchromatosis

pigmentation, abnormal: chloasma,
chromatism, chromatosis,
hyperpigmentation,
hypopigmentation, jaundice,
melanosis, melasma

pigment-bearing cell: chromatophore

pigment production: chromatogenous,
chromogenesis

pigment secretion: chromocrinia

piles: hemorrhoids

pill: anovulatory drug, bolus, capsule,
lozenge, medication, medicine, oral
contraceptive, pastille, pellet,
pharmaceutical, physic, placebo,
tablet, troche

pimple: papulo-, boil, carbuncle,
comedo, furuncle, milium, papilla,
papule, pustule, wheal

pin: dowel

pincers: forceps

pinch: constrict

pineal body disorder: pinealism,
pinealopathy

pineal body surgery: pinalectomy

pineal body tumor: pinealoma,
pineoblastoma

pine cone shaped: pineal, piniform

pink disease: acrodynia, erythredema
polyneuropathy

pinkeye: conjunctivitis

pink puffer: chronic obstructive
pulmonary disease

pinprick sensation: acanthesthesia,
acmesthesia

pinworm: Enterobius vermicularis,
Oxyuris

pinworm disease: enterobiasis,
oxyuriasis

pit: alveolus, antrum, cavity,
depression, faveolus, fossa, fovea,
furrow, hiatus, lacuna, lamina,
pockmark, scrobiculus, sinus

pitcher-shaped: urceiform

pit formation: umbilication

pitted: alveolate, carious, scrobiculate

pituitary gland: hypophysis,
hypophysis cerebri,
neurohypophysis

pituitary gland, frontal lobe:
adenohypophysis

pituitary gland diseases: acromegaly,
acromicria, Cushing's disease,
diabetes insipidus, dwarfism,
dyspituitarism, eunuchoidism,
Frohlich's syndrome, gigantism,
hyperpituitarism, hypogonadism,
hypopituitarism,
panhypopituitarism, pituitarism,
Sheehan's syndrome, Simmond's
disease

pituitary gland inflammation:
hypophysitis

pituitary gland removal: apituitarism,
hypophysectomy

pituitary gland tumors: acidophilic
adenoma, craniopharyngioma,
eosinophilic adenoma, Nelson's
syndrome

pivot: axis

place: topo-, locus, zone

place, fear of: topophobia
placental detachment: abruptio
placentae
placental disorders: accreta, previa,
spuria
placental inflammation: placentitia
placental-like: placentoid
placental tumor: placentoma
places, fear of high: acrophobia
plague: pestis, Yersinia
plague therapy: antilemic
plan: regimen
plant: phyto-
plantar wart: verruca plantaris
plaque: atheroma
plasma deficiency: anhydremia,
oligoplasmia
plastic: acrylic, polyvinyl chloride,
Silastic
plastic surgery: -plasty, alloplasty,
anaplasty, autoplasty,
chalinoplasty, geniocheiloplasty,
genioplasty, genitoplasty,
genyplasty, morioplasty,
rhinoplasty, rhytidectomy
See also specific tissues
plastic surgery procedure:
retrenchment
plate: denture, lamella, lamina,
platelet
platelet abnormality: thromboasthenia
platelet disintegration:
thrombocytolysis
platelet formation: thrombocytopoiesis,
thrombopoiesis
platelet production: thrombopoiesis
platelets, decreased:
thrombocytopenia, thrombopenia
platelets, increased: polyplastocytosis,
thrombocythemia, thrombocytosis
pleasure: hedonism
pleasure, decreased: hyphedonia
pleasure, fear of: hedonophobia
pleasure, lack of: anhedonia
pleasure principle: hedonism
pleura, arising in: pleurogenous

pleura, wash out: pleuroclysis
pleura adhesions: pleurodesis
pleura bleeding: pleurorrhagia
pleura cavity, air in: pneumatothorax,
pneumothorax
pleura cavity, pus in: pyohemothorax
pleura diseases: aeropleura,
aerothorax, pneumatothorax,
pneumohemothorax,
pneumohydrothorax,
pneumopyothorax,
pneumoserothorax, pneumothorax,
pyohemothorax, pyopneumothorax,
pyothorax
pleura hernia: pleurocele,
pneumatocele
pleura inflammation: corticopleuritis,
empyema, parapleuritis, pleurisy,
pleuritis, pleurocholecystitis,
pleurohepatitis, pleuropericarditis,
pleuropneumonia,
pneumoperitonitis
pleura inspection: pleuroscopy
pleura pain: pleuralgia
pleura surgery: pleurectomy,
pleurocentesis, pleuroparietopexy,
pleurotomy, thoracocentesis,
thorocentesis
pliable: resilient
pliers: extractor, forceps
pluck: extract
plug: pledget, stype, tampon
pock: blister, pustule
pocket: cavity, fissure, orifice, pouch,
sac
pockmark: cicatrix
point: punctum
pointed: acerate, acuminate, ensiform,
sagittal, xiphoid
points, anatomical: acanthion,
antinion, aromion, asterion,
auriculare, basion, bregma, clition,
condylion, dacryon, entomion,
genion, glabella, gnathion, gonion,
infradentale, inion, jugale,
jugomaxillary, koronion, lambda,
McBurney's, nasion, obelion,
ophryon, pogonion, porion,
prosthion, pterion, rhinion,

salpingion, sphenion, staphylion,
staurion, stenion, stephanion,
subnasal, symphysion, tylion,
tympanion, zygion
pointlike: punctiform
points, fear of: aichmophobia
poison: toxi-, toxico-, toxo-, echidnin,
endotoxin, exotoxin, histotoxin,
toxenzyme, toxin, venom
poison, affinity for: toxophil
poison, craving for: toxicomania
poison, diseases from: toxemia,
toxicoderma, toxicodermatitis,
toxicopathy, toxicosis, toxidermitis,
toxipathy, toxonosis
poison, fear of: toxicophobia,
toxiphobia
poison, science of: biotoxicology,
toxicology
poison antidote: alexipharmac,
antitoxin, toxicide, toxicosozin,
toxolysin, toxophylaxin
poison carrying: veneniferous
poison containing: toxiferous
poison immunity: mithridatism
poisoning: allantiasis, amphetamines,
barbiturates, benzene, berylliosis,
botulism, bromide, carbon dioxide,
carbon monoxide, carbon
tetrachloride, cyanide, DDT,
decarborane, diborane, emetism,
ergotism, formaldehyde,
galactotoxism, gasoline,
hydrofluoric acid, hydrogen sulfide,
ichthyism, ichthyosarcotoxism,
kerosene, lead, lye, mercury,
methane, methyl ethyl ketone,
muscarine, mycetismus,
mytilotoxism, nicotine, nitric acid,
nitrobenzine, opiates, oxygen,
ozone, pentaborane,
phenothiazines, phosgene,
platinum, ptomaine, salicylates,
salmonellosis, silver, totuene,
urosepsis, venenous, veneration,
vinyl chloride, virose, zinc,
zincalism, zootrophotoxis

poisoning, fear of: iophobia,
toxicophobia
poison ivy: Rhus dermatitis
poisonlike: toxicoid, toxoid
poison oak: Rhus dermatitis
poisonous, excessively: hypertoxicity
poisonous, slightly: hypotoxicity
poison producing: toxicogenic,
toxigenic, venenific
poison removal: detoxification
poisons, as therapy: toxicotherapy
poison specialist: toxicologist
poison sumac: Rhus dermatitis
poison tablets: toxitabellae
poliomyelitis preventive: Sabin
vaccine, Salk vaccine
pollute: contaminate
polyp: polypus
polyp, of nose: rhinopolypus
polyp disease: polyposis
polyplike: polypoid
polysaccharides: agar-agar,
carbohyrate, cellulose, dextrin,
disaccharide, glycogen, gum arabic,
hemicelluose, hexopentosan,
hexosan, inulin, monosaccharide,
pectin, pentosan, starch
poor: mal-
porcupine disease: ichthyosis
porous: absorbent, cancellous,
perforated, permeable, polyporous
porphyrin disease: porphyria
portal vein: pyle-
portal vein dilation: pylephlebectasis
portal vein inflammation: pylephlebitis
portal vein occlusion: pylemphraxis,
pylethrombosis
portend: prognosis
portion: aliquot, pars, segment
portly: obese
port-wine stain: birthmark, nevus
flammeus
positions: Alvert's, anatomic,
Bozeman's, Brickner's, Caldwell,
decubitus, Depage's, Elliot's,
English, Fowler's, Fuchs, lithotomy,
Mayer, prone, Robson's, Rose's,
Simon's, Sims, site, situs, supine,
Titterington, Trendelenburg,
Valentine's, Walcher, Waters

positive: an-, ana-, adient
positive pole, toward: anaphoresis
possessing: -ate
posterior: dorsi-, dorso-, caudal,
   dorsal, gluteal
postmortem: autopsy, necropsy
potassium, deficient: hypokalemia,
   hypopotassemia
potassium, excessive: hyperkalemia,
   hyperpotassemia
potassium in blood: kalemia
potassium in urine: kaliuresis
potency, fear of losing: aphanisis
potency, lack of: agenesis, impotence
pouch: bursa, cavity, sac, saccule,
   saccus, utricle, ventricle
pouch, blind: caecus, cecum, cul-de-sac
pouch formation: marsupialization
poultice: cataplasm, fomentation,
   mustard plaster, plaster, sinapism
poultice-like: pultaceous
pound: beat, palpitate, pulse,
   pulverize, throb
poverty, fear of: peniaphobia
powder: pulvis, trituration
powderlike: pulverulent
power: dynamo-, potency
power, reduced: adynamic, asthenic,
   attenuated, impotent
pox: chickenpox, smallpox, syphilis,
   varicella, variola, venereal disease
preceding: ante-, pro-, precursor
precipices, fear of: cremnophobia
prediction: prognosis
predisposition: diathesis, susceptibility
pregnancy: conception, cyesis,
   cyophoria, enciente, encyesis,
   gestation, gravidism, impregnated,
   inseminated, monocyesis, obstetric,
   para, parturient, syllepsis,
   uterogestation
pregnancy, abdominal: abdominocyesis
pregnancy, absence: acyesis
pregnancy, before: progravid
pregnancy, diagnosis: Ascheim-Zondek
   test, ballottement repercussion,
   bitterling, Friedman test, rabbit
   test

pregnancy, extrauterine:
   abdominocyesis, cornual, eccyesis,
   ectopic, metacyesis, oocyesis,
   ovariocyesis, tubal
pregnancy, false: phantom pregnancy,
   pseudocyesis, pseudopregnancy
pregnancy, first: unigravida, unipara
pregnancy, mask of: chloasma
   gravidarum
pregnancy, multiple: bipara, duipara,
   multigravida, multipara,
   octigravida, octipara, plurigravida,
   pluripara, quadripara, quartipara,
   quintipara, secundipara,
   septigravida, septipara,
   sextigravida, sextipara, tripara
pregnancy, poisoning: eclampsia,
   preeclampsia, toxemia
pregnancy, terminated: aborted,
   miscarriage
pregnancy complication: sphenosis
pregnancy division: trimester
pregnancy preventive: cervical cap,
   coil, coitus interruptus, condom,
   diaphragm, diethylstilbesterol,
   intrauterine device, oral
   contraceptive, pessary, rhythm
   method, sponge, tubal ligation,
   vasectomy
premature: precocious, rudimentary,
   vestigial
prenatal diagnosis: amniocentesis,
   fetoscopy, ultrasonography
preparation: concoction, drug,
   medication, medicine,
   pharmaceutical
prepuce, absence: aposthia
prepuce inflammation: acrobystitis,
   acroposthitis, posthitis
prescription: drug, formula, medicine,
   pharmaceutical, recipe, remedy
presentation, abnormal: asynclitism,
   breech, brow, crossbirth, footling,
   Litzmann's obliquity, Naegele's
   obliquity, transverse
press together: coarctate, compression,
   constrict

pressure: baro-
pressure, equal: isotonic
pressure, internal: eccentropiesis
pressure sensitive: piesthesia
pressure sore: decubitus ulcer
pretend: malinger, simulate
preventive: prophylactic, vaccine
prick: perforate, puncture
prickling: paresthesia
prickly heat: lichen tropicus, miliaria
    rubra, tropical lichen
primal: embryonic, genetic, germinal,
    nascent
primary: paleo-, protopathic
primate: biped, mammal, man
principal: arch-, arche-, archi-
probe: examination, radiolus, sound
procedure: maneuver, method,
    operation, protocol, technique,
    treatment
procedure, standardized: protocol
process: -asis
process, constructive: anabolism
process, destructive: catabolism
process, fingerlike: digitation
producing: -genesis, -genic, -ferous,
    -poietic
progressive: degenerative, malignant
projection: acantha, apophysis,
    condyle, cyst, denticle, eminence,
    excrescence, node, papilla,
    processus, prominence, promontory,
    tooth, tuberosity, tumor, villus
prolapse: -ptosis, ptosis
proliferate: metastasize
prominence: acantha, apophysis,
    condyle, cyst, denticle, eminence,
    excrescence, node, processus,
    projection, promontory, tooth,
    tuberosity, tumor, villus
propagate: disseminate, reproduction
propensity: diathesis
prophylactic: condom, vaccine
prostate calculus: prostatolith
prostate discharge: prostatorrhea
prostate disease: prostathelcosis,
    prostatism, prostatosis

prostate enlargement: prostatauxe,
    prostatomegaly
prostate excision: prostatectomy,
    prostatomyomectomy,
    prostatovesiculectomy, prostectomy
prostate incision: prostatocystotomy,
    prostatomy, prostatotomy
prostate inflammation: prostatitis,
    prostatocystitis, prostatovesiculitis
prostate pain: prostatalgia,
    prostatodynia
prostate surgery: prostatolithotomy
prostate ulceration: prostatelcosis
prosthesis: artificial limb, denture,
    hearing aid, pacemaker
prostrate: prone, supine
prostration: neurasthenia, neurosis,
    psychophysiologic asthenic reaction
protected: immune
protective: esophylaxis, immunization,
    phylaxis, vaccine
protein, developing from:
    proteinogenous
protein, excessive: hyperproteinemia,
    hyperproteosis
protein, fear of: proteinophobia
protein breakdown: albuminolysis,
    proteolysis
protein fixation: proteopexy
protein in blood, excessive:
    proteinemia
protein in tissue, excessive: proteinosis
protein in urine, excessive:
    albuminuria, proteinuria, proteuria
protein producing: proteinogenous
prothrombin, in blood:
    prothrombinemia
prothrombin deficiency:
    hypoprothrombinemia,
    prothrombinopenia
protoplasm: axoplasm, cytoplasm,
    hyaloplasm, hyalotome,
    nucleoplasm
protoplasm mass: cenocyte, syncytium
protozoa: Amoeba, Babesia,
    Balantidium, Cryptosporidium,
    Entamoeba, Giardia, Iodamoeba,
    Isospora, Leishmania, Plasmodium,

Pneumocystis, Sarcocystis,
Toxoplasma, Trichomonas,
Trypanosoma
protozoan diseases: amebic dysentery,
amebiasis, babesiosis, balantidiasis,
Chagas disease, coccidioidomycosis,
coccidiosis, cryptosparidiosis,
giardiosis, isosporiasis, malaria,
sleeping sickness, toxoplasmosis,
trichomoniasis
protozoan therapy: antiprotozoa
protrusion: hernia
protuberance: apophysis, condyle, cyst,
excrescence, mons, monticulus,
node, nodosity, outgrowth, process,
projection, prominence, swelling,
tumor
proud flesh: granulation tissue
psoas inflammation: psoitis
psoriasis preventive: antipsoriatic
psyche: psych-, psycho-, ego, id,
personality, superego
psychiatric disciplines: biologic,
orthopsychiatry, psychoanalysis,
psychobiology
psychiatric disorder: *See* mental
diseases
psychiatric techniques: autocatharsis,
catharsis, group psychotherapy,
psychoanalysis, psychocatharsis,
psychodrama, psychotherapy
psychiatric therapies: antidepressants,
antipsychotics, electroconvulsive,
gelotherapy, psychosurgery
psychoanalysis patient: analysand
psychologic disciplines: analytic,
applied, experimental, Jungian
psychologic therapies: assertiveness
training, aversion, behavior
modification, biofeedback,
desensitization, family, group,
operant conditioning, reciprocal
inhibition
psychosis: anergasia
puberty, study of: ephebology
puberty changes: adrenarche

puberty onset: pubarche, pubertas
pubic: pubo-, pubio-
pubic bone: pecten
pubis surgery: pelviotomy, pubiotomy
pudendal apron: tablier
puffiness: edema
pull: adduct
pulling: traction
pull out: abarticulated, dislocated,
extract
pully-shaped: trochlea
pulmonary: *See also* lung
pulmonary valve: semilunar valve
pulp: chyme, marrow
pulp inflammation: pulpitis
pulsate: systaltic
pulsation: beat, palpitate, palpitation,
throb
pulse: sphygmo-, sphygmus
pulse, abnormal: acrotism, anacrotic,
anadicrotism, asphyctic, bisferious,
bounding, Corrigan, dicrotic,
hemisystole, intermittent,
paradoxical, pulsus parvus
pulse, rapid: pyknocardia, tachycardia
pulse, slow: bradycardia, bradycrotic,
bradyrhythmia, bradysphygmia
pulseless disease: Takayasu's arteritis
pulselike: sphygmoid
pulse pressure measurement:
sphygmobolometry,
sphygmography
pulse tracing: catacrotism,
catadicrotism, catatricrotism,
dicrotic notch
pump: Abbot, breast, Harvard, heart,
infusion, insulin, oxygenator,
stomach
puncture: cente-, centesis, incision,
nyxis, paracentesis, perforation,
trephine
puncture, abdominal:
abdominocentesis, amniocentesis,
celiocentesis, enterocentesis,
paracentesis
pungent: acrid, caustic

punishment, fear of: poinephobia
pupil: core-, -coria, coro-, pupillo-
pupil, absent: acorea
pupil, artificial: coremorphosis,
    coretomedialysis
pupil, between: interpupillary
pupil, double: dicoria
pupil abnormality: corectopia,
    dyscoria, polycoria, triplokaria
pupil closure: corecleisis, iridencleisis,
    synezesis
pupil constrictor: acetylcholine
    chloride, miotic
pupil contraction: miosis
pupil destruction: corelysis
pupil dilation: corectasia, corediastasis,
    mydriasis, platycoria
pupil dilator: atropine, cyclopentolate,
    homatropine, mydriatic,
    phenylephrine, scopolamine,
    tropicamide
pupil disorder: Adie's syndrome,
    asthenocoria, hippus
pupil excision: corectomy, iridectomy
pupil incision: coretomy, iridotomy
pupil narrowing: corestenoma, miosis,
    stenocoriasis
pupil occlusion: corecleisis
pupils, equal: isocoria
pupils, unequal: anisocoria
pupil surgery: corectomedialysis,
    coredialysis, coreoplasty,
    coroparelcysis
pure: antiseptic, homozygous,
    sterilized
purgative: aperient, cathartic, clyster,
    enema, ipecac, laxative
purify: cleanse, depurant, rectify,
    sanitize, sterilize
purifying: abstergent
purple blindness: anianthinopsy
purulent: pus, gangrenous, gleet,
    sanies, suppuration, ulceration,
    vomicose
pus: py-, pyo-, abscess, archepyon,
    emphyema, gleet, ichor, leukorrhea,
    purulence, pustule, pyecchysis,
    pyemia, sanies, septicemia,
    suppurate

pus, spitting: pyopytsis
pus, spreading of: pyoplania
pus, swallow: pyophagia
pus accumulation: pyocele
pus cell: leukocyte
pus discharge: pyorrhagia, pyorrhea
pus diseases: pyoderma,
    pyodermatitis, pyodermia
pus formation: empyesis, purulent,
    pyogenesis, pyopoiesis, suppuration
pus formation preventive:
    antipyogenic
pus in abdomen: pyocelia
pus in blood: pyemia, pyotoxinemia,
    septicemia, suppurative fever
pus in cavity: abscess, empyema
pus in cranium: pyocephalus
pus in cyst: pyocyst, pyopneumocyst
pus in ear: pyolabyrinthitis,
    pyotorrhea
pus in eye: hypopyon, pyophthalmia,
    pyophthalmitis
pus in fallopian tube: pyosalpinx
pus in feces: pyochezia, pyofecia
pus in gallbladder:
    pyopneumocholecystitis
pus in heart: pyopericarditis,
    pyopneumopericardium
pus in joint: pyarthrosis
pus in lung: empyema
pus in ovary: pyoovarium,
    pyosalpingitis, pyosalpingo-
    oophoritis
pus in peritoneal cavity:
    pyoperitoneum, pyoperitonitis,
    pyopneumoperitonitis
pus in pleural cavity: pyohemothorax
pus in semen: pyospermia
pus in seminal vesicles: pyovesiculosis
pus in urachus: pyourachus
pus in ureter: pyoureter
pus in urine: colipyuria, pyoturia,
    pyuria
pus in uterus: pyometra,
    pyophysometra
pus in vagina: pyocolpocele, pyocolpus

puslike: puriform, puruloid, pyoid
pus treatment: pyotherapy
pustule: abscess, carbuncle, chancre, comedo, furuncle, hordeolum, milium, papilla, ulceration, wen
pustule eruption: pustulosis
putrefaction: gangrene, mortification, necrosis, saprogenic, sphacelus
putrid: sapro-
pylorus displacement: pyloroptosis
pylorus examination: pyloroscopy
pylorus inflammation: pyloroduodenitis, pyloritis
pylorus narrowing: pyloristenosis, pylorostenosis
pylorus spasm: pylorospasm
pylorus surgery: pylorectomy, pylorogastrectomy, pyloromyotomy, pyloroplasty, pylorostomy, pylorotomy

Q

quack: charlatan
quake: ictus, jactitation, oscillate, seizure, shake, stroke, tremble, waver
quality of: -acu
qualm: anxiety, nausea
queasy: dizzy, faint, nauseous
quench: satiate, suppress
quickening: fetal movement
quicksilver: mercury
quiescent: comatose, dormant, immobile, inactive, inertia, latent, lethargic, stagnant, torpid
quiet: anechoic
quinsy: peritonsillar abscess
quirk: aberration, anomaly, fetishism, monomania, obsession
quiver: convulse, fibrillate, flutter, oscillate, palpate, pulsate, shiver, throb, tremble, tremor, undulate
quotidian: amphemerous, malaria

R

rabbit fever: tularemia
rabbit test: Friedman test
rabies: lysso-, hydrophobia, lyssa, Negri bodies, rabid
rabies, fear of: cynophobia, hydrophobophobia, lyssophobia
rabieslike: rabiform
rabies preventive: antilyssic, antirabic
race history: phylogeny
racking: acute, painful
radiant: phosphorescent
radiation: actin-, actino-, radio-
radiation-caused diseases: actinotoxemia, radiocystitis, radiodermatitis, radioepidermitis, radioepithelitis, radionecrosis, radioneuritis, radiotoxemia
radiation disease, study of: radiopathology
radiation emission: radio-, radioactive
radiation measurement: dosimetry
radiation producing: actinogenic, radiogenic
radiation specialist: radiologist, roentgenologist
radiation therapy: actinopraxis, actinotherapy, radiopraxis, radiotherapy
radiology, shadow: adumbration
ragged: serrated
raging: delirious, furibund, furious, hysterical, maniacal
rain, fear of: ombrophobia
raises: elevator, levator
rale, hissing: sibilus
rally: convalesce, recuperate
ramus inflammation: ramitis
ramus surgery: ramicotomy, ramisection
rancid: mephitic
rapid: tachi-, tacho-, tachy-

rare: atypical
rash: -anthema, efflorescence,
    eruption, erythema multiforme,
    exanthema, lesion, roseola
    See also skin rash
rasping sound: sibilate, stertorous
rat bite fever: spirillum fever
rat bite infection: sodoku
rational: sane
raving: delirious, hysterical, irrational
raw: excoriated, macerated, skinned
ray: actino-, emanation, irradiation,
    radiation
reaction: allergy, anaphylactic, hay
    fever, hives, hypersensitivity
reaction, peculiar: idiosyncrasy
reactive: resistant
reading disability: alexia,
    anagnosasthenia, bradylexia,
    dyslexia, strephosymbolia
rear: buttocks, fundament, posterior
reasoning, disordered: paralogia
rebirth: catharsis
rebound: reflux
recede: abate, retrograde
recent: ceno-, neo-
recipe: formula, prescription
reciprocal: repercussion
reclining: decubitus, prone, supine
recollection: anamnesis
recombine: anastomose, splice
reconstruction: plastic surgery
recovery: analepsis, convalescence,
    reactivation, recuperate,
    reintegration
rectum: archo-, proct-, procto-, recto-
rectum, fear of: proctophobia,
    rectophobia
rectum bleeding: archorrhagia,
    proctorrhagia
rectum dilation: proctectasia
rectum discharge: archarrhea,
    proctorrhea
rectum diseases: colitis, hemorrhoids,
    imperforate anus, proctopolypus,
    prolapse

rectum examination:
    proctocolonoscopy, proctoscopy,
    proctosigmoidoscopy
rectum excision: proctocolectomy,
    prolectomy, rectectomy,
    rectosigmoidectomy
rectum fistula: archocystocolposyrinx,
    archocystosyrinx
rectum fixation: proctococcypexy,
    proctopexy, proctosigmoidopexy,
    rectococcypexy, rectopexy,
    romanopexy, sigmoidopexy
rectum hernia: archocele, proctocele,
    rectocele
rectum incision: proctocystotomy,
    proctotomy, proctovalvotomy,
    rectocystotomy
rectum inflammation: colproctitis,
    paraproctitis, proctitis,
    proctocolitis, proctosigmoiditis,
    rectitis, rectocolitis
rectum infusion: proctoclysis,
    rectolysis
rectum narrowing: archostenosis,
    proctostenosis, rectostenosis
rectum pain: proctagra, proctalgia,
    proctodynia, rectalgia
rectum paralysis: proctoparalysis,
    proctoplegia
rectum prolapse: archoptoma,
    archoptosis, proctoptosis
rectum spasm: proctospasm, tenesmus
rectum specialist: proctologist
rectum surgery: proctocolpoplasty,
    proctocystoplasty,
    proctoperineoplasty, proctoplasty,
    proctorrhaphy, proctostomy,
    proctotoreusis, rectoplasty,   ·
    rectorrhaphy, rectostomy
recumbent: clinostatism, decubitus,
    prone, reclining, supine
recuperate: convalesce, recover
recurrence: cycl-, cyclo-, pali-, palin-,
    chronic, palindromia, recidivism,
    recrudescence, relapse
red: erythro-, rhodo-, ruber,
    rubescent, rubrum, sanguine

red, fear of: erythrophobia
red blindness: anerythropsia,
daltonism, erythropsia, protanopia,
xanthocyanopsia
red blood cell: erythroblast,
erythrocyte, hematocyte,
reticulocyte
red blood cell, abnormal: achromocyte,
burr, echinocyte, helmet,
microspherocyte, poikilocyte,
schistocyte, schizocyte, spherocyte
red blood cell, immature: erythroblast,
macroblast, megaloblast, neocyte,
proerythroblast, promegaloblast,
reticulocyte
red blood cell, large: macrocyte,
megaloblast, megalocyte
red blood cell, nucleated: pyrenemia
red blood cell, spiny: acanthocyte
red blood cell clumping:
hemagglutination
red blood cell deficiency: anemia,
erythropenia, oligocythemia,
oligocytosis, oligoerythrocythemia
red blood cell destruction:
erythrocytolysis,
erythrocytophagy,
erythrocytorrhexis,
erythrocytoschisis, erythrolysis,
erythrophagia, erythrorrhexis,
hematocytolysis, homolysis, isolysis,
plasmorrhexis, plasmotropism
red blood cell diseases:
anisopoikilocytosis,
erythroblastosis, erythrocytosis,
erythropathy, favism, microcytosis,
rhestocythemia
red blood cell formation:
erythrogenesis, erythropoiesis
red blood cell formation, lack of:
anerythroplasia
red blood cells, excessive: erythremia,
erythrocythemia, erythrocytosis,
hypercythemia, polycythemia,
polycythemia vera
red faced: florid, plethora

red gum: strophulus
red-haired: erythrism
redirect: anastomosis, shunt
red marrow: bone marrow
redness: eosin, erythema, florid, flush,
ruber, rubiosis
red skin: plethora, rubefacient
red spot: spiloplaxia
red-staining, easily: erythrophile
reduced: deoxy-, desoxy-, -lysis,
plication
reel foot: See clubfoot
reeling: staggering, titubation
referred pain: synalgia
refined: distilled
reflection: anaclasis, clone, replication
reflex, absent: areflexia
reflex, decreased: hyporeflexia
reflex, increased: hyperreflexia
reflex action: anaclasis
reflexes: abdominal, Achilles tendon,
anal, appendical, arc, attention,
attitudinal, audito-oculogyric,
auditory, auriculocervical,
auriculopapebral, autonomic,
Babinski, Bainbridge, Bechterew's,
biceps, blink, bregmocardiac,
Brissauds, bulbocavernous,
bulbomimic, cardiac,
cardiovascular, cat's eye,
Chaddock's, chain, chemoreflex,
ciliary, ciliospinal, clasp-knife,
cochleo-orbecular, conditioned,
conjunctival, consensual,
contralateral, convulsive, corneal,
corneomandibular, cremasteric,
cry, defecation, digital, direct,
doll's eye, dorsal, elbow, embrace,
epigastric, Erben's, Escherich's, eye
closure, facial, faucial, front-tap,
gag, gastrocolic, gastroiliac,
Gault's, Geigel's, Gifford's,
Hoffmann, jerk, Kisch's, light,
micturation, Moro, nasolabial, neck
righting, nostril, obliquus, patellar,
Piltz's, plantar, rectal, righting,
scapulohumeral, sexual, sneeze,
Snellen's, startle, statotonic,
stretch, superficial, tendon, triceps,

tympanic, unconditioned,
vagovagal, vascular, vesicle, virile,
viscerosensory, zygomatic
reflexes, instrument for measuring:
anacamptometer
reformation: neogenesis
refracture: anaclasis
refuse: detritus, phytodetritus,
residue, tartar biodetritus,
zoodetritus
regeneration: epimorphosis,
neogenesis, reproduction,
textoblastic
regimen: diet, method, therapy,
treatment
regress: recur, reflux, relapse, subside
regular: chronic, periodic, quotidian,
recurring, rhythmic
regurgitation: reflux
rejection preventive: antilymphocytic
serum, azathioprine,
betamethasone, chlorambucil,
corticotropin, cyclophosphamide,
cyclosporine, dexamethasone,
hydrocortisone,
immunosuppressives,
mercaptopurine, paramethasone,
prednisolone, prednisone,
triamcinolone
rejuvinate: cell therapy,
organotherapy, revive, resuscitate
relapse: degenerate, palindromia,
recidivisn, recrudescence,
recurrence, regress, retrocession,
retrogression
relax, inability to: achalasia
relaxing: anetic
relieve: -lysis, abirritate, analeptic,
analgesic, emollient, palliative,
sedative, tranquilizer
religion, fear of: hierophobia
religious mania: theomania
remainder: dedritus, residue, residuum
remedies, study of: acognosia
remedy: analgesic, anodyne,
antibiotic, antitoxin, cathartic,
drug, embrocation, emollient,
medication, medicine, palliative,
pharmaceutical, prescription,
purgative, sedative, therapy,
tranquilizer, treatment, unguent,
vaccine
remedy, secret: arcanum
remissions: polyletpic
removal: -ectomy, ablate, abscission,
amputation, apheresis, aspirate,
biopsy, clearance, debridement,
desquamation, excision, exfoliation,
extirpation, obliterate, resection
removing: amotio
renal tubule: nephron
renewal: recurrence, regeneration,
rejuvenation, relapse, resuscitation
rent: cleft, crevice, fissure, fracture,
incision, interstice, lacerate,
perforation, puncture, rupture,
tear
repair: cure, heal, regenerate
repeated: recurrent
repellent: apocrustic, fetid, nauseating
repetition: pali-, palin-, tauto-,
duplication, perseveration,
replication
replacement part: prosthesis
report: case history
repose: dormant, inactive, inanimate,
latent
representative: -type, class
repression: inhibition
reproach, fear of: enissophobia
reproduction: conception, duplication,
fertilization, procreation,
replication
reproduction, science of: genesiology
reproductive cell: gamete, gonocyte,
ovum, spermatozoon
reproductive organs: genitalia, testes,
vas deferens, prostate, seminal
vesicles, urethra, penis, ovary,
fallopian tubes, uterus, vagina,
vulva
repulsive: fetid, nauseating, noxious
resembling: -oid, quasi-, -ular
reservoir: cisterna
residue: detritus

resilience: elasticity, flexibility
resistance: immunity, impedance,
    obstruction
resistance, lack of: susceptibility
resistance mechanism: immunology
resistant: refractory, rigidity
resonance: tympanitic
resonance increased: hyperresonance
resorption: lysis
respiration: pneum-, pneuma-,
    pneumato-, air, anapnea,
    breathing, eupnea, pneusis
respiration, abnormal: apnea, apneusis,
    asphyxia, Biot's, Bouchut's,
    Cheyne-Stokes breathing, chokes,
    dyspnea, hyperpnea,
    hyperventilation, hypopnea,
    hypoventilation, oligopnea,
    orthopnea, panting, pneusis,
    polypnea, tachypnea
respiration, noisy: stridor
respiratory diseases: asphyxiation,
    asthma, bronchiectosis,
    bronchiolitis, bronchitis,
    bronchopneumonia, catarrh, croup,
    hyaline membrane disease,
    influenza, pneumoconiosis,
    pneumonia, silicosis,
    tracheobronchitis, tuberculosis
respiratory disease treatment:
    atmiatrics, bronchodilators,
    oxygen, ventilation
respiratory movements, measurement
    of: spirography
respiratory stimulants: aminophylline,
    theophylline
respiratory system: nasal cavity, upper
    respiratory tract (pharynx, larynx,
    trachea), lower respiratory tract
    (bronchi, bronchioles, lungs),
    diaphragm
respiratory tract examination:
    bronchoscopy, spirometry
response: hypersensitivity reaction
responsibility, fear of:
    hypengyophobia

resting: dormant, lethargy, sopor,
    static, stupor, torpor
resting stage: interphase, telogen
restlessness: agitation, akathisia,
    dysphoria, hyperprogia
restoring: analeptic, refection,
    regeneration, rehabilitation,
    repair, resuscitation, tonic
restraint: brace, camisole, corset,
    obstruction, straightjacket
restricted: localized
result: -asis
retarded: See mental retardation
retch: vomiturition
retention: continence, memory
reticular-like: cancellous
reticulocytes, decrease:
    reticulocytopenia, reticulopenia
reticulocytes, increase: reticulocytosis
reticuloendothelial cells: clasmatocyte,
    histiocyte, macrophage, microglia,
    Kupffer cell, splenocyte
reticuloendothelial system diseases:
    follicular lymphoma, fungoides,
    Gaucher's disease, Hodgkin's
    disease, lymphosarcoma, mycosis,
    Niemann-Pick disease, reticulum
    cell sarcoma
retina: amphiblestrodes, cones, pars
    ciliaris, pars iridica, pars optica,
    ora serrata, rods
retina bleeding: Eales' disease
retina diseases: detachment,
    maculopathy, neuroretinopathy,
    photoretinitis, retinopathy,
    retrolental fibroplasia
retina examination:
    electroretinography, retinoscopy
retina image, equal: isocoria
retina image, prolonged: afterimage,
    photogene
retina inflammation: amphiblestritis,
    neuroretinitis, papilloretinitis,
    retinitis, retinochoroiditis,
    retinopapillitis
retina-like: retinoid

retina pigment: chromophane
retina regeneration: rhodophylaxis
retina softening: retinomalacia
retina surgery: hydrodictiotomy
retina swelling: albedo retinae
retina tumors: dictyoma, diktyoma,
    retinoblastoma, retinocystoma
retraction: abduction, anastole
retrogression: catagenesis,
    degeneration, disintegration,
    relapse
return: recurrence, relapse
reversal: allo-, dis-, un-
reversion: atavism, regression, relapse
revert back: atavism, paleogenesis,
    retrogression
revive: anabiosis, regenerate,
    rejuvenate, resuscitate
revolve: gyrate, pivot, trochoid
rheumatism: arthritis
rheumatism therapy: antirheumatic
rhythm variation: arrhythmia,
    cacorhythmic, dysrhythmia
rib: cost-, costi-, costo-, pleur-,
    pleuro-, costa, pleurapophysis
rib excision: costectomy,
    costotransversectomy,
    thoracectomy
rib fixation: costopneumopexy
rib incision: costotomy
ribless: ecostate
riblike: costiform
rib pain: costalgia, pleurodynia
ribs, between: intercostal
rib surgery: costosternoplasty,
    pleuropneumonolysis
ricelike: riziform
rickets causing: rachitogenic
richets therapy: antirachitic
rickettsia diseases: Brill's disease, Q
    fever, rickettsialpox, rickettsiosis,
    Rocky Mountain spotted fever, tick
    fever, trench fever, typhus
rid: catharsis, elimination
rider's bone: adductor muscle
    concretion, cavalry bone

ridge: loph-, bridge, carina, crest,
    crista, edge, fold, pilaster, plica,
    rachis, raphe, rim, ruga
ridicule, fear of: categelophobia
rift: aperture, cavity, cleft, crevice,
    fissure, lacuna, orifice
right: dextr-, dextro-, dextral
right, fear of: dextrophobia
right-eyed: dextrocular, dextrocularity
right-handed: dextral, dextromanual
right side, toward: dextrad
right turning: dextroduction,
    dextrogyrate, dextrorotatory,
    dextrotropic, dextroversion
rigid: hard, immobile, inflexible, tense
rigidity: acampsia, ankylosis, erection,
    rigor mortis
rim: border, brim, crest, edge, margin,
    ridge, vallate
ring: crico-, gyro-, annular, annulus,
    areola, band, circle, corona, disk,
    fold, globule, gyrate, zone
ringing in ears: tinnitus
ring-shaped: cricoid
ringworm: tinea
Rio Grande fever: brucellosis
rip: lacerate, rupture
ripe: mature
ripening: maturation
risk: vulnerable
river blindness: onchocerciasis
rivers, fear of: potamophobia
robbers, fear of: harpaxophobia
rod: rhabdo-
rodent ulcer: Jacob's ulcer,
    Krompecker's tumor
rods, fear of: rhabdophobia
rod-shaped: bacilliform, baculiform
roll: -volute, convolute, involution,
    vortex
rolled up: volute
roof of mouth: palate
root: radi-, rhizo-, radicle, radicular,
    radix
rootlike: radiciform, radicle, rhizoid,
    rhizome

root surgery: rhizodontrypy, rhizotomy
rope-shaped: filiform, restiform
rose-colored: roseo-, flushed
rose fever: pollinosis, rhinitis
roselike: rosette
rot: sapro-, decomposition, gangrene, mortification, necrosis, putrefaction, putrescence, putrid, suppuration
rotate: gyrate, pivot, trochoid
rotate inward: pronate
rotate outward: extorsion
rotund: fat, obese
rough: villous
roughage: fiber
round: cycl-, cyclo-, disk
roundworm: Acanthocheilonema, Ancylostoma, Ascaris, Brugia, Capillaria, Dipetalonema, Dracunculus, Enterobius, Filaria, Loa, Mansonella, Necator, nematodes, Onchocerca, Strongyloides, Toxocara, Trichinella, Trichuris, Wuchereria
roundworm diseases: acanthocheilonemiasis, ancylostomiasis, aniskiosis, ascariasis, capillariasis, dipetalonemiasis, dracunculiasis, enterobiasis, erythrasma, filariasis, larva migrans, mansonelliasis, nectoriasis, nematodiasis, onchocerciasis, strongyloidiasis, toxocariasis, trichinosis, wuchereriasis
roundworm preventive: ascaricide
rub: chafe, embrocation, massage
rubber: condom
rubbing: frottage, inunction, paratripsis, perfrication
    See also massage
rubbing treatment: grattage
rub off: abrade, plane
ruddy: flushed, sanguine
rudiment: anlage, primordium, vestige

ruination, fear of: atephobia
rumbling in intestines: borborygmus
rump: buttocks, gluteal region
run: effluence, flow, flux
runaround: felon, panaris, paronychia
run forward: procursive
runner's knee: chondromalacia, patellalgia
runny nose: coryza, hydrorrhea
runs: diarrhea
run together: coalesce, confluent
rupture: -clasis, break, cleft, fissure, fracture, hernia, rhegma, rhexis
rust: oxidize
rust-colored: rubiginous
rut: canal, channel, fossa, furrow, stria

S

sac: cyst-, cysti-, cystido-, cysto-, bladder, bleb, blister, bursa, capsule, cavity, crypt, cyst, follicle, loculus, pouch, saccule, saccus, vesicle
sac, abnormal: diverticulum
sac, blood vessel: aneurysm
saclike: sacciform
saclike structure: acinus, alveolus
sacroiliac joint inflammation: sacrocoxitis, sacroiliitis
sacroiliac joint pain: sacrocoxalgia
sacrum: sacro-
sacrum, long: dolichohieric
sacrum pain: hieralgia, sacralgia, sacrodynia
sacrum surgery: sacrectomy, sacrotomy
saddle back: lordosis
saddle-shaped: sella
sadness: depression, melancholia
sag: concave, curvature, ptosis, sway back
Saint Anthony's fire: erysipelas
saliva: ptyalo-, sial-, sialo-, ptsyma, sialine, slaver, sputum

saliva, decreased: aptyalia, asialia, hypoptyalism, hyposalivation, oligoptyalism, oligosialia, sialaporia, xerostomia

saliva, excessive: hygrostomia, hypersalivation, ptyalism, ptyalorrhea, salivation, sialism, sialorrhea

saliva, excessive swallowing: sialaerophagia, sialophagia

saliva, loss of: sialozemia

saliva analysis: sialosemeiology

saliva flow: sialosis

saliva inducer: ptyalagogue, sialogogue

saliva producing: sialogenous

saliva reducer: antisialagogue, antisialic, atropine

salivary duct dilation: sialectasia

salivary duct inflammation: angiosialitis, sialitis, sialoangiitis, sialodochitis

salivary duct narrowing: sialostenosis

salivary ducts: Bartholin's, parotid, Rivinus, sublingual, submandibular

salivary duct surgery: sialodochoplasty

salivary duct tumor: ptyalocele, sialoncus

salivary gland: sialaden

salivary gland calculus: ptyalith, ptyalolith, sialolith, tophus

salivary gland disease: cytomegalic inclusion disease

salivary gland examination: ptyalography, sialography

salivary gland fistula: sialosyrinx

salivary gland inflammation: hyposialadenitis, sialadenitis, sialitis, sialoadenitis

salivary glands: buccal, parotid, sublingual, submaxillary

salivary gland secretion: cerumen, sebum, smegma

salivary gland surgery: ptyalolithotomy, sialadenectomy, sialoadenotomy, sialolithotomy

salivary gland tumors: sialadenoncus, sialocele

salivary vomiting: sialemesis

saliva suppression: sialoschesis

salt: sodium chloride

salt removal: desalination

salts: cathartic, Epsom, laxative, potassium, purgative, Rochelle

salty: brine, saline

salve: abirritant, anodyne, balm, cerate, demulcent, embrocation, emollient, lenitive, liniment, magma, ointment, palliative, unguent

same: homeo-, homoeo-, homoio-, ipsi-, tauto-

same side: homolateral, ipsilateral

sample: biopsy, specimen

sand bath: ammotherapy, psammotherapy

sandlike: arenoid

sandy: acervulus, arenaceous, granular, gritty, psammous, sabulous, tophaceous

sane: rational

sanguine: bloodlike, feverish, flushed, rubescent, rubicund, ruddy, sunburned

sanitary: antiseptic, aseptic, decontaminated, disinfected, hygienic, prophylactic, sterile

sanitary napkin: menstrual pad, perineal pad, tampon

satiety: -coria, saturation

satisfied: replete

saturation: -rhaphy, permeation

sausage-shaped: allantoid, botuliform

saw-toothed: crenated, dentated, serration

scab: crust, eschar

scab formation: incrustation

scabies, fear of: scabiophobia

scabies therapy: antiscabietic

scablike: incrusted, psoriatic

scabs, multiple: squarrose

scald: ambustion

scald head: tinea favosa
scale: lepido-, lamella, lamina, layer, plate, squama
scalelike: furfuraceous, lamellar, scute, squamous, squarrose
scalenus surgery: scalenectomy, scalenotomy
scalloped: crenated
scalp: epicranium, napex
scalp bleeding: cephalhematoma
scalp disease: scutulum
scalp inflammation: scall
scaly diseases: impetigo, pityriasis, psoriasis
scan: computed tomagrophy, nuclear magnetic resonance, probe, ultrasonography
scapula projection: acromion
scapula surgery: scapulectomy, scapulopexy
scar: ule-, ulo-, cautery, cicatrix, epulosis, escharotic, keloid, pit, pockmark, rhagade
scar formation: cicatrization
scar formation, stimulating: cicatrizant, synulotic
scar incision: cicatricotomy, ulotomy
scarlet fever test: Dick test
scarlike: uloid
scarlike formation: cicatrization, ulosis
scar removal: chemabrasion, cicatrectomy, dermabrasion, ulectomy
scar surgery: y-plasty, z-plasty
scar tumor: keloid
scattered: diffuse, dispersion, disseminated, dissipated
sciatic nerve inflammation: ischiatitis
science of: -ology
sclera disorder: sclerophthalmia
sclera inflammation: episcleritis, leucitis, logaditis, scleritis, sclerochoroiditis, scleroticochoroiditis, sclerotitis
sclera protrusion: sclerectasia, staphyloma

sclera softening: scleromalacia
sclera surgery: sclerectomy, scleriritomy, scleronyxis, scleroplasty, sclerostomy, scleroticectomy, scleroticonyxis, scleroticopuncture, scleroticotomy, sclerotomy
scourage: pestilence, plague
scrape: abrasion, burn, chafe, curettage, friction, laceration, puncture, raclage, rasura, wound
scratched, fear of being: amychophobia
scrawny: cachectic, cadaverous, emaciated, gaunt, skeletal
scrotum: oscheo-, osheal
scrotum, urine in: urocele, uroscheocele
scrotum disease: chylocele, chyloderma, hydrocele, rhacoma
scrotum excision: scrotectomy, varicocelectomy
scrotum hernia: scrotocele
scrotum inflammation: oscheitis, oschitis, scrotitis
scrotum surgery: oscheoplasty, scrotoplasty
scrotum tumor: oscheocele, oscheoma, oscheoncus, steatocele
scrub: abstergent
scrub typhus: tsutosugamushi
scruff: nape, nucha
scurf: dandruff
scurvy preventive: antiscorbutics, ascorbic acid (vitamin C)
sea, fear of: thalassophobia
seam: cicatrix, commissure, furrow, junction, raphe, ridge, scar, sutura
seasick: See motion sickness
seat: buttocks, gluteus, nates
seatworm: pinworm
sebaceous gland calculus: sebolite, smegmolith
sebaceous gland diseases: asteatosis, stearoderma, steatocryptosis, steatopathy, steatosis
sebaceous gland disease-producing: steatogenous

sebaceous gland excretion, excessive:
seborrhagia, seborrhea
sebaceous gland inflammation:
thylacitis
sebaceous gland secretion: cerumen,
sebum, smegma
sebaceous gland tumor: steatadenoma
sebum: cerumen, smegma
sebum-producing: sebiparous
secluded: isolated, quarantined
second cranial nerve: optic
second sight: gerontopia, senopia
secretion, abnormal: dyscrinism,
hypersecretion, parasecretion
secretion, absent: acrinia, amyxia
secretion absorbent: desiccant,
exsiccant
secretion-causing: crinogenic,
secretagogue
secretion change: diacrisis
secretion increase: sialogogue,
succorrhea
secretions, inability to retain:
acathexia
secretions, study of: crinology
secretion suppression: apolepsia
sectioned: cutting, incision, merotomy,
segmentation
securing: fixation, immobilization,
suturing
sedatives: adinazolam, alonimid,
alprazolam, amobarbital, analgesic,
anodyne, aprobarbital, barbiturate,
bentazepam, benzoctamine,
butabarbital, butalbital, calmative,
chloral betaine, chloral hydrate,
chlordiazepoxide, chlorpromazine,
cloperidone, clorazepate, clorethate,
clozapine, cyrazepam, dexclamol,
diazepam, diphenhydramine,
doxylamine, ethchlovynol,
ethinamate, etomidate, fenobam,
flurazepam, glutethimide,
halazepam, hexobarbital,
hydroxyzine, hypnotic, lorazepam,
lormetazepam, mecloqualone,
mephobarbital, meprobamate,
mesoridazine, methaqualone,
methyprylon, midaflur, narcoleptic,

narcotic, nisobamate, nitrazepam,
opiate, oxazepam, palliative,
paraldehyde, pentobarbital,
phenobarbital, prazepam,
prochlorperazine, promethazine,
propiomazine, pyrilamine,
quazepam, reclazepam,
secobarbital, soporific, suproclone,
talbutal, temazepam, thalidomide,
thioridazine, tracazolate,
tranquilizer, trepipam, triazolam,
tricetamide, triclofos,
trifluoperazine, triflupromazine,
trimeprazine, trimetozine,
uldazepam, zolazepam
sedentary: dormant, immobile, sessile
sediment: fecula, hypostasis,
precipitate, residue, residium
seduction: nymphomania, satyriasis
seed: gono-, gamete, germ, ovum,
primordium, semen, sperm,
spermatozoon, zygote
seen, by naked eye: gross
seen, fear of being: scopophobia
seepage: discharge, defluxion, effusion,
exudation, secretion, transudation
seizing: prehension
seizure: -lepsia, -lepsis, -lepsy,
apoplexy, attack, convulsion,
epilepsy, grand mal, ictus,
paraxysm, petite mal, raptus,
stroke
self: aut-, auto-, consciousness, ego,
personality, psyche
self-centered: egocentric, narcissistic
self-controlling: autonomic
self-destructive disease: autoimmune
disease, suicide
self-interest, abnormal: egomaniac
self-love: autoeroticism, autophilia,
narcissism
self-nourishing: autotrophic
self-poisoning: autotoxemia
self-preoccupation: introversion
self-production: autogenesis,
autogenous

self-restraint: continence
self-understanding: insight
semen: gon-, gono-, ejaculate, seminal fluid
semen, pus in: pyospermia
semen abnormality: aspermia, spermacrasia, spermatopathia
semen discharge: ejaculation, emission, spermatism
semen excretion, in urine: semenuria, seminuria, spermaturia
seminal calculus: spermolith
seminal fluid: semen
seminal fluid disorder: polyspermia
seminal inflammation: spermatocystitis
seminal vesicle: gonecyst, spermatocyst
seminal vesicle, pus in: pyovesiculosis
seminal vesicle calculus: gonecystolith
seminal vesicle examination: vesiculography
seminal vesicle inflammation: gonecystitis, spermatocystitis, vesiculitis
seminal vesicle surgery: spermatocystectomy
semiprone: Sims position
senile: anile, senescence
senility: Alzheimer's, senilism
senility, premature: Hutchinson-Gilford syndrome, progeria
sensation: esthesio-, affect, esthesia
sensation, abnormal: acanthesthesia, allochiria, anesthesis, atopognosia, dyschiria, dysesthesia, formication, hemidysesthesia, hemihyperesthesia, hemihypesthesia, heteresthesia, paraphia, parapsia, paresthesia, phonism, photism, pseudesthesia, pseudochromesthesia, synchiria, synesthesia
sensation, absence: acroanesthesia, agnosia, anesthecinesia, anesthesia, paralysis

sensation, acute: algesia, hyperesthesia, hyperpathia, hypersensitivity, oxyesthesia, oxypathia
sensation, return of: palinesthesia
sensation conducting: sensiferous
sensation perception: cheirognostic, chirognostic
sense organ: chemoreceptor, neuron
senses: hearing, sight, smell, taste, touch
senses, abnormally sharp: hyperacuity
senses, normal: eucrasia, euesthesia
sensitivity test: scratch
separate: crin-, asymphytous, bisect, discrete, precipitate
separation: ap-, apo-, dis-, ablation, abruptio, detachment, diastasis, dissepiment, dissociation, divergence
separation, forceful: dis-, avulsion
septum: septulum
septum surgery: septectomy, septostomy, septotomy
serious: acute, critical
serotonin inhibitors: cinanserin, fenclonine, fonazine, mianserin, pizotyline, xylamidine
serous membrane: pericardium peritoneum, pleura
serous membrane inflammation: orrhomeningitis, serositis
serpentine: sinuous
serrated: crenate, denticulate
serum: orrho-, sero-
serum, antibody in: antiserum
serum, study of: orrhology, serology
serum reaction: orrhoreaction, seroreaction
set: fixation
seventh cranial nerve: facial
seven-year itch: scabies
sever: amputate, bifurcate, bisect, divulse, sement
several: multi-, pluri-, poly-
severe: acute, fatal, mortal

sewing: ligature, suture
sex: gender
sex, lack of: asexual
sex, opposite: heterosexual
sex, same: homosexual
sex, study of: sexology
sex act: a tergo, coitus, concubitus,
    copulation, ejaculation, fellatio,
    fornication, intercourse, onanism,
    pederasty, sodomy
sex activity, periodic: estrus
sex cells: gameto-, gamete, ovum,
    spermatozoon
sex cells, kills: gametocide
sex cells, maturation: gametogenesis,
    oogenesis, spermatogenesis
sex change: transsexual, viraginity
sex characteristics, lack of:
    defeminization, demasculinization
sex drive: libido
sex drive, abnormal: anaphrodisia,
    gynecomania, lascivia,
    nymphomania, satyriasis
sex hormones, lack of: agenitalism
sex instinct: eroticism
sexless: asexual
sex organs: clitoris, genitals, gonads,
    labia majora, labia minora,
    muliebria, penis, pudendum,
    scrotum, testes, vagina, virilia
sex organs, abnormal: agonadal,
    androgynous, anorchia, dysgonesis,
    gynander, gynandrous,
    hermaphroditism, hypogenitalism,
    hypogonadism, microgenitalism,
    pseudohermaphroditism
sex organs, diseases: See genital
    diseases, venereal diseases
sex organs, removal of: asexualization,
    castration, ovariectomy, vasectomy
sexual abnormalities: algolagnia,
    anedeous, anilinction, anorthosis,
    antaphrodisiac, anthropophagy,
    aphrodisiomania, autoeroticism,
    bestiality, bisexual, buggery,
    coprolagnia, cunnilingus, eonism,
    erotomania, erotopathy,
    exhibitionism, flagellation,
    frigidity, frottage, hyperovaria,

iconolagny, impotence, incest,
    irrumation, lecheur, lust,
    masochism, mixoscopia, narcissism,
    necrophilia, necrosadism,
    nympholepsy, paraphilia,
    pederasty, pederosis, pedophilia,
    peotillomania, perversion,
    premature ejaculation,
    pseudomasturbation, renifleur,
    sadism, sapphism, scapophilia,
    sexual anesthesia, sodomy,
    transvestism, tribadism, troilism,
    urolagnia, voyeur, zoolagnia,
    zooerastia, zoophilism
sexual climax: orgasm
sexual desire: eroto-, amativeness,
    aphrodisia, eroticism, libido
sexual development, premature:
    hyperovaria
sexual excitement, producing:
    erogenous, erotogenic
sexual gratification: manustupration,
    masturbation
    See also sex act
sexual intercourse, abnormality:
    apareunia, dyspareunia
sexual love, fear of: coitophobia,
    cypridophobia, erotophobia
sexual potency, fear of losing:
    aphanisis
sexual preferences: asexual, bisexual,
    heterosexual, homophile,
    homosexual, lesbian, sapphism
sexual reproduction: amphigony
shadow: ghost corpuscle, phantom
    corpuscle
shaft: diaphysis, duct, scapus, support,
    tube
shaggy: hirsute
shaking: convulsion, chorea, palsy,
    paralysis, quassation, tremble,
    vibration
shaking palsy: paralysis agitans,
    Parkinson's disease
shape: -morph, form
shape, abnormal: paramorphia

shapeless: amorphous, anidean
shapes, multiple: multiform, polymorphous
sharp: acerate, acrid, acute, lancinating, xiphoid
sharp objects, fear of: belonephobia
shaving: tonsure
sheath: theco-, theca, capsula, integument
sheaths, between: intervaginal, intrathecal
sheaths, within: intraspinal, intrathecal
shed: deciduous, desquamate, exfoliate, molt, slough
sheet: lamina, plate
shell: calix, cavity, cortex
shell-shaped: thyreo-, thyro-, conchoidal, scutiform
shell shock: combat neurosis, hysteria
shin: cnemis
shinbone: shank, tibia
shingles: herpes zoster
shin splints: medial tibial syndrome
shiver: shaking, tremor
shock: anaphylaxis, cardiogenic, electric, hypovolemic, insulin, psychic, trauma
shoe support: patten
short: brachy-, brevi-, steno-
shorten: contract
shortening: contraction, retraction
shortness of breath: dyspnea
shortsighted: myopia, hypometropia
shot: angle, view
shoulder: omo-, scapulo-, clavicle and scapula, acromion
shoulder bandage: scapulary
shoulder blade: scapula
shoulder blade, between: interscapilium, interscapulum
shoulder disease: omagra
shoulder inflammation: omarthritis, omitis
shoulder ligament: glenohumeral
shoulder muscles: deltoid, subscapularis, teres

shoulder pain: omalgia, omodynia, scapulalgia, scapulodynia
shoulder paralysis: neuralgic amyotrophy
shoulder socket: glenoid cavity
shrink: atrophy, contract
shrivel: atrophy, dehydrate, desiccate, kraurosis, waste away
shudder: convulsion, paroxysm, spasm, tremor
shuffle: dragging gait, limp
shunt: bypass
shut in: confine, convalescent, introverted, invalid, quarantine, valetudinarian
shutting: obturation, occlusion, synizesis
Siamese twins: parabiosis
See also twins, conjoined
sick: ill, nauseous
sickle cell anemia: meniscocytosis
sickle-shaped: crescent, falcate, falciform, falx
sickly: cachetic, invalid, valetudinarian
sickness: affection, cachexia, disease, disorder, dysfunction, ideopathy, infection, morbidity, pathology
sick-to-stomach: motion sickness, nausea, vomiting
side: latero-, lateral
side-by-side: apposition, contiguity, juxtaposition
sievelike: cribrate, cribriform, ethmoid
sigh: exhale, expire, suspiration
sight: -blepsia, -blepsy, opto-, vision
See also eye
sigmoid colon inflammation: sigmoiditis
sigmoid colon surgery: cecosigmoidostomy, sigmoidectomy, sigmoidopexy, sigmoidoproctostomy, sigmoidorectostomy, sigmoidostomy, sigmoidotomy

sign: indication, symptom, trait
sign language: cheirology, dactylology,
    signing
silent: aphonia, mute, still
similar, in function: analog
similar to: -an, homeo-, homoeo-,
    homoio-, -ian
similar structure: homologous,
    homology, homoplastic
simple: herb
simultaneous: concomitant, isochronal,
    synchronous
sinew: tendon
sinewy: fibrous
singe: cauterize
single: haplo-, mon-, mono-, uni-,
    azygos
single-celled: monocellular,
    monolocular
single-minded: monobulia, monoideism,
    monomania
sinuous: anfractuous, convoluted
sinus examination: sinography
sinus inflammation: aerosinusitis,
    barosinusitis, pansinusitis,
    perisinusitis, polysinusitis, sinuitis,
    sinusitis
sinuslike: sinusoid
sinus surgery: sinuotomy, sinusotomy
sisters and brothers: siblings
site: locus
sit still, inability to: akathisia, restless
    legs syndrome
sitting, fear of: kathisophobia
sixth cranial nerve: abducens
size, excessive: acromegaly, gigantism
size, increase: hyperplasia,
    hypertrophy
size, reduced: hypoplasia, hypotrophy
size reduction: hyperinvolution,
    plication, superinvolution
skeletal diseases: achondroplasia,
    Albright's disease, ankylosing
    spondylitis, rickets
skeleton: skeleto-, bony framework
    See also bone

skin: derma-, dermat-, dermato-,
    -dermia, -dermic, dermo-, corium,
    cuticle, cutis, dermis, epidermis,
    integument, peau, pellicle, pore,
    stratum corneum, stratum
    germinativum, stratum
    granulosum, stratum lucidum,
    tegumen
skin, abscessed: dermapostasis
skin, absence: adermia
skin, beneath: hypodermic,
    subcutaneous, subcuticular,
    subdermal, subepidermal,
    subepithelial
skin, blue-colored: cyanoderma,
    cyanopathy, cyanosis,
    hypercyanosis
skin, bone in: osteodermia, osteosis
    cutis
skin, break in surface: excoriation
skin, burning sensation: uredo,
    urtication
skin, crawling sensation: formication
skin, dead: exfoliation, scale, slough
skin, dimpled: peau d'orange
skin, hair, nails: dermoskeleton,
    exoskeleton, integumentary
    system
skin, scaly: ichthyosis
skin, scraped: excoriation
skin, smooth: leiodermia
skin, study of: dermatology,
    dermatopathology, dermonosology
skin, through: endermic, percutaneous,
    transdermal
skin, within: intradermal
skin abnormality: adermogenesis
skin abrasion: contusion, excoriation,
    laceration, rhacoma, wound
skin atrophy: anetoderma
skin bleeding: dermatorrhagia,
    petechiae
skin burn: blister, scald, sunburn
skin coloration: chloasma, lividity,
    macule, melanin, melanoderma,
    melanoleukoderma, melanopathy

skin coloring agents: dyes, psoralen,
stains, tar, trioxsalen
skin cyst: dermatocyst
skin cyst excision: dermoidectomy
skin darkening: tanning
skin discoloration: argyria, argyrism,
argyrosis, dermatokelidosis,
dyschroa, dyschromia, ecchymosis,
ephelis, erythrosis, freckle, lentigo,
livedo, macula, melanoderma,
melanosis, pelioma, peliosis,
poikiloderma, purpura, roseola,
sideroderma, spiloplaxia, tache,
urticaria pigmentosa, vitilipoidea,
xanthelasmoidea, xanthochromia,
xanthoma, xanthoderma
pigmentosum, xanthosis
skin disease, fear of: dermatophobia
skin diseases: acanthosis nigricans,
angiokeratoma, angiolupoid,
arevareva, blue nevus, chloracne,
condyloma, cutis marmorata,
dermamyiasis, dermatoneurosis,
dermatopathy, dermatosclerosis,
dermatosis, dermographia,
dermomycosis, dermopathy,
elastoma, epidermosis,
erythrokeritodermia, furunculosis,
genodermatosis, geroderma,
Gougerot-Carteaud syndrome,
Haber's syndrome, hyperkeratosis,
hystriciasis, ichthyosis, impetigo,
intertrigo, keratoacanthoma,
keratoderma, keratonosis,
keratosis, kerion, leiodermia, lichen,
molluscum, morphea,
neurodermatosis, orf,
parakeratosis, parapsoriosis,
pemphigus, phymatosis, pityriasis,
pseudoacanthosis nigricans,
pseudoxanthoma, psora, psoriasis,
pyoderma, rhus dermatitis,
ringworm, Ritter's disease,
rosacea, scabies, scall, scleroderma,
scrofuloderma, seborrheic
dermatitis, steatocystoma

multiplex, steatomatosis,
toxicoderma, trichophytid,
urtication, xanthomatosis
skin disease test: Wood's rays
skin dryness: xeroderma, xeronosus,
xerosis
skin eruption: arthritide, bromoderma,
epidermophytid, exanthem,
exanthema subitum, exanthesis,
hives, hydroa, miliaria,
phyrnoderma, rash, roseola
infantum, urticaria
skin examination: dermatoscopy
skin fissures: rhagades
skin grafting: dermatoautoplasty,
dermatoplasty, epidermization
skin growth: acrochardon,
cuticularization, epidermoma, spur
skin hardening: callosity, callus,
sclerema, scleriasis
skin hypertrophy: chalazoderma, cutis
laxa, dermatauxe, dermatocele,
dermatolysis, dermatomegaly,
elephantiasis, epidermolysis,
pachydermatocele
skin induration: acroscleroderma,
sclerodactylia, scleroma
skin infections: acladiosis,
ancylostomiasis, boil, carbuncle,
cellulitis, chromoblastomycosis,
chromomycosis, dermatomycosis,
dermophlebitis, dermatophytosis,
ecthyma, epidermomycosis,
erysipelas, furuncle, impetigo,
neurodermatitis, pyodermatitis,
tinea
skin inflammation: acne,
acrodermatitis, actinodermatitis,
berlock dermatitis, contact
dermatitis, dermatitis,
dermatomucosomyositis,
dermatomyositis, dermatophytid,
eczema, epidermitis, erysipelas,
erythema nodosum,
haplodermatitis, intertrigo,
keratodermatitis, lichen planus,
photodermatitis, radiodermatitis,
radioepidermitis, sclerodermatitis,

staphylodermatitis,
streptodermatitis,
toxicodermatitis, ulodermatitis
skin injury: bruise, contusion,
laceration, wound
skin irritation: chafing,
dermatoconiosis, itch, pruritus
skin layers: stratum corneum, stratum
lucidum, stratum granulosum,
stratum germinativum
skin lesion: stigma, stigmatization,
ulcer
skinlike: dermoid
skin of head: scalp
skin pain: dermalgia, dermatalgia,
dermatodynia, erythralgia
skin parasite: dermatophyte
skin patch: plaque
skin pigment, absence: achromasia,
achromia, achromoderma, albinism,
cafe-au-lait, hypopigmentation,
leukasmus, leukoderma,
leukopathia, pseudoalbinism,
vitiligo
skin producing: dermatogenesis
skin reaction: cutireaction
skin redness: erubescence, erythema,
erythroderma, flare, florid, flush,
plethora, rubefaction, rubor
skin scale: furfur
skin scratches: scarification
skin secretion, excessive: dermatorrhea
skin shedding: dandruff,
desquamation, ecdysis, exfoliation,
keratolysis, sloughing
skin softener: emollient
skin softening: dermalaxia
skin specialist: dermatologist
skin spot remover: emaculation
skin surgery: dermatoplasty
skin test: Mantoux, Schick, scratch,
Tzanck
skin therapy: dermatotherapy
skin thickening: acanthosis,
dermatoma, keratosis,
lichenification, pachyderma,
pachydermatosis

skin tightener: astringent, styptic
skin tumors: acanthoma,
angiokeratoma, basal cell nevus,
Degos' disease, dermatofibroma,
dermatofibrosarcoma protuberans,
dermatomyoma, glomangioma,
mycosis fungoides, papilloma,
phyma, pilomatricoma, tuberous
carcinoma, trichoepithelioma,
tubulodermoid
skin wrinkling: rhicnosis
skin writing: graphesthesia
skull: crani-, cranio-, calvaria,
cranium, occiput, sinciput
See also cranium, face, head
skull, abnormal: brachycephaly,
craniostosis, phenozygous,
plagiocephaly
skull, broad and high:
hypsibrachycephalic
skull, flat: tapinocephaly
skull, high and pointed: oxycephalia
skull, large: macrocephaly,
megalocephaly, platystencephaly
skull, long: dolichocephalic
skull, narrow: stenocephaly
skull, short: brachycephaly
skull, study of: craniology,
craniometry, phrenology
skull, thick: pachycephaly
skull bone removal: cephalotrypesis,
trephination
skull bones: frontal, temporal,
parietal, occipital, sphenoid,
ethmoid, nasal, lacrimal, inferior
nasal concha, zygomatic, maxilla,
mandible, palatine, vomer
skullcap: calvaria
skull covering: endocranium,
epicranium, scalp
skull defect: clinocephaly
skull fissure: diastematocrania
skull fracture: contrafissure, gutter
skull protuberance: inion, mastoid
process
skull puncture: craniopuncture

skull softening: craniomalacia, craniotabes

skull surgery: craniectomy, cranioplasty, craniotomy, trephining

skull union: sutura, suture, synarthrosis

slack: flaccid, limp

slanting: abaxial, oblique

slapped cheek disease: erythema

slash: incision, laceration, rupture, wound

sleep: hypno, somn-, somni-, somno-, coma, dreams, hallucination, hibernation, hypnotism, nonrapid eye movement, rapid eye movement, sleepiness, somnolence, sopor, trance

sleep, fear of insomnia: agrypniaphobia

sleep, study of: hypnology

sleep, talk in: somniloquism

sleep diseases: dysphylaxia, hypersomnia, insomnia, Kleine-Levin syndrome, narcolepsy, parahypnosis, somnipathy

sleep inducers: hypnogenetic, hypnogogue, hypnotic, sedative, somnifacient, somniferous, soporific

sleeping sickness: encephalitis, encephalitis lethargica, hypersomnia, hypnolepsy, narcolepsy, nona, trypanosomiasis

sleeplessness: agrypnia, ahypnia, ahypnosis, insomnia, vigil, wakefulness

sleeplike: soparose

sleeplike state: catalepsy, coma, hypnosis, trance

sleep preventive: agrypnotic, anthypnotic, antihypnotic

sleep producing: *See* hypnotics, sedatives

sleep state: hibernation, hypnotized, nonrapid eye movement, predormition, rapid eye movement

sleep walking: noctambulism, paroniria ambulans, somnambulism

slender: lepto-

slice: section

slimy: myx-, myxo-, uliginous

sling: brace

sling-shaped: fundiform

slipped: dislocated, prolapsed

slipped disk: herniated intervetebral disk

slippery: lubricated, mucoid, synovial, unctuous

slit: aperture, cleft, crack, fissure, incisure, rima, rimula

slope: clivus, gradient, oblique

slough: eschar

slough removal: escharotomy

slow: brady-, dull, retarded, subside

slow onset: insidious

sluggish: indolent, inert, lethargic, phlegmatic, somnolent, torpid

slur: sibilate

small: micr-, micro-, nano-, olig-, oligo-, -ule, -ulum

smallpox: variola

smallpox, mild: alastrim, amaas, variola minor

smallpox eruption: alices, pustules

smallpox innoculation: variolation

smallpox-like: varioloid

smart: ache, pain, sting, throb

smegma calculus: smegmolith

smell: osmo-, aroma, cacosmia, effluvium, fetid, fetor, mephitic, odor, odorant, odoriferous, odorivector, olfact, olfaction, osmesis, parosmia, putrid, rancid, stench

smell, acuteness: oxyosmia, oxyrhine

smell, absence: anodmia, anosmia, anosphrasia

smell, eroticism of: osmolagnia, osphresiolagnia

smell, measurement: odorimetry

smell, study of: olfactology, osmology, osphresiology

smell defect: hemianosmia, hyposmia,
  merosmia
smell disorders: dysosmia, parosmia,
  parosphresia, pseudosmia
smell of feet: podobromidrosis
smell sense: olfaction, osphresis,
  rhinesthesia
smoker's tongue: leukoplakia
smooth: leio-, depilated, glabrous
smother: asphyxiate, envelope, extinct,
  suffocate
snail fever: schistosomiasis
snake poisoning: ophidism,
  ophiotoxemia
snakes, fear of: ophidiophodia
snap: fracture
sneeze causing: sternutator,
  sternutatory
sneezing: ptarmus, sternutatio
sniff: inhale
sniffer: renifleur
snore: stertor
snow blindness: niphablepsia,
  niphotyphlosis
soak: infuse, permeate, saturate
soap: sapo, saponaceous
society, fear of: apanthropia
socketlike: glenoid
sodium in blood, decreased:
  hyponatremia
sodium in blood, excessive:
  hypernatremia, natremia
sodium in urine, decreased:
  antinatriuresis
sodium in urine, excessive: natriuresis
soft: ductile, flaccid, flexible,
  gelatinous, malleable, pia, pliable,
  semiliquid
soften: macerate
softening: malacia, mollities
soft palate: velum palatinum
soft sore: chancroid
soft spot: fontanelle
soft tissue, study of: sarcology
soft tissue decomposition: sarcolysis
soft tissues: flesh, muscles

soil: contaminate, pollute
soiling: encopresis, enuresis
solar plexus: celiac plexus
solar therapy: heliotherapy
sole: azygous, volar
sole of foot: plantar, thenar
solid: stereo-, clotted, coagulated,
  compressed, condensed, congealed,
  dense, inspissated
solids: capsule, confection, extract,
  lamella, lozenge, ointment, plaster,
  powder, pill, suppository, tablet
solitude, abnormal desire for:
  agromania
solution: lyo-, decoction, dilution,
  emulsion, fluid extract, infusion,
  liniment, mixture, suspension,
  tincture
solvent: medium, menstruum, vehicle
sonogram: ultrasonography
sonorous: pulsating, resonant,
  vibrating
sooth: palliate, tranquilize
soothing: abirritant, anetic, balm,
  calmative, demulcent, lenitive,
  obtundent, palliative, relaxing
sore: abscess, ache, inflamed,
  irritation, laceration, leproma,
  lesion, pain, pustule, ulcer, wound
sore, painful: canker
sore, painless: chancre
sore throat: laryngitis, quinsy,
  sphagitis, staphyloangina,
  staphylococcal infection,
  streptoangina, streptococcal
  infection, tonsillitis
sorrow: grief
sort: genus, species, strain, variety
soul: anima
sound: audio-, phon-, phono-,
  acoustics, amphorophony,
  articulation, auscultation, bruit,
  click, crackles, crepitations,
  healthy, hyperphonesis,
  hypophonesis, murmur,
  pectorophony, pectoriloquy,
  pelgaphonia, rales, rational, rattle,

resonance, snoring, souffle,
strepitus, vocalization
See also speech
sound, fear of: acousticophobia,
phonophobia
sound, involuntary: aboiement
sound, loud: sonorous
sound, memory loss for:
acousmatamnesia
sound, remote: micracusia
sound, science of: phonetics, phonology
sound, splashing: clapotage, succussion
sound echo: reverberation
sound hallucinations: acousma
sound of fluid in cavity: hydatism
sound sensitivity: hyperacusis
source: genesis
sourness: -oxy, acescence, acetic, acor
space: areola, camera, cavitas, cavity,
cavum, hiatus, loculus, vacuole,
vestibule
space, empty, fear of: cenophobia,
kenophobia
Spanish collar: paraphimosis
spare: auxiliary
sparkling: scintillation
sparse: sporadic
spasm: -clonia, spasmo-, clonus,
convulsion, eclampsia, epilepsy,
ictus, jactitation, orgasm,
paroxysm, seizure, spasmus,
tetany, throe, tic
spasmodic: arrhythmic
spasm producing: spasmogenic
spasm prone: spasmophilia
spasm reliever: antispasmodic,
spasmolytic
spasm termination: spasmolysis
speak: articulate, talk
speaking, fear of: laliophobia
speaking in tongues: glossolalia
specific: diacritic
specimen: biopsy, culture, slide
speck: ephelis, granule, lentigo,
particle
spectacles: *See* eyeglasses

spectrum: spectro-, infrared, invisible,
visible, ultraviolet
speech: lalo-, logo-, Broca's area,
phone
See also voice
speech, excessive: leresis, lalorrhea,
logorrhea, polyphrasia,
verbomania, volubility
speech, inability to understand:
acatamathesia, asemia
speech, meaningless: allophasis,
divagation, embolalia, embololalia,
embolophrasia, idioglossia,
schizophasia, verbigeration
speech, obscene: coprotalia
speech, rapid: agitolalia, agitophasia,
oxylalia, tachylabia, tachyphrasia
speech, slow: baryglossia,
bradyglossia, bradylalia,
bradyphrasia
speech, soundless: endophasia
speech, unintelligible: lallation
speech abnormalities: aprosody,
barylalia, betacism, cluttering,
dysphonia, echolalia, heterolalia,
heterophasia, heterophemia,
inarticulate, labialism, logagnosia,
laloneurosis, lambdacism, lisp,
logognosia, logoklony, logomania,
logopathia, mogiphonia, palilalia,
paralambdacism, pararhotacism,
parasigmatism, pyknophrasia,
rhotacism, scanning, sigmatism,
staccato
speech defects, study of: logopedics
speech disability: acataphasia, alogia,
aphemia, aphthongia, gammacism,
motor aphasia
speech diseases: aglossia,
agrammatism, alalia, allolalia,
alogia, anarthria, angophrasis,
anomia, aphasia, asyllabia,
ataxaphasia, cataphasia,
dysarthria, dyslalia, dysphasia,
dysphrasia, hypologia,
jargonophasia, lalopathy,
logoclonia, logopathy, logospasm,
mogilalia, motor aphasia, mutism,
olophonia, paliphrasia,

paragrammatism, paralalia,
paralexia, paraphasia, paraphrasia,
perseveration, phonopathy,
psellism, smudging, spasmophemia,
stuttering, syllabic
speech loss: alalia, alogia, anarthria,
aphroma
speech organs, paralysis of: logoplegia
speed: amphetamine
spell: duration, hypnotism,
mesmerism, period
sperm: spermo-, spermato-, acrosome,
ejaculate, gamete, germ cell,
semen, spermatozoon
sperm, absence: aspermatism,
aspermia, azoospermia,
oligospermia
sperm, decreased: spermatocrasia
sperm, fear of losing: spermatophobia
sperm, immature: spermatid,
spermatoblast, spermoblast
sperm, loss of: spermatocrasia,
spermatorrhea
sperm abnormality: dyszoospermia,
necrospermia
spermatic cord: funiculus
spermatic cord disease: mumu
spermatic cord inflammation:
chorditis, corditis, funiculitis,
perispermatitis, spermatitis
spermatic cord obstruction:
spermatemphraxis
spermatic cord pain: spermoneuralgia
spermatic cord surgery: funiculopexy
spermatic cord vein, enlargement:
pampinocele, varicocele
sperm cell: androgone
sperm destruction: spermatocidal,
spermatolysis, spermatotoxin,
spermicidal, spermotoxin
sperm development: spermatogenesis
sperm disease: spermatopathy
spermlike: spermatoid
sperm suppression: spermatoschesis
sphenoid bone incision: sphenoidotomy
sphenoid bone inflammation:
sphenoiditis

sphere: sphero-, globulus, globus, orb,
spherule
sphincter ani pain: sphincteralgia
sphincter inflammation: sphincteritis
sphincter spasm: sphincterismus
sphincter surgery: sphincterectomy,
sphincteroplasty, sphincterotomy
spider: arachn-, arachno-
spider bite poisoning: arachnidism,
arachnoidism
spike: spicule, spiculum
spiky: acantho-
spin: gyration, rotation
spinal canal, air in: pneumatorrhachis
spinal column: *See* vertebral column
spinal cord: myel-, myelo-, pyramidal
tract
spinal cord, absence: amyelencephalia,
amyelia
spinal cord, away from: spinifugal
spinal cord, small: micromyelia
spinal cord abnormality:
diastematomyelia,
myeloradiculodysplasia,
myeloschisis, rachischisis,
syringomyelocele
spinal cord atrophy: amyelotrophy,
myelanalosis, myelophthisis
spinal cord bleeding: hematomyelia,
myelapoplexy, myelorrhagia
spinal cord defects: atelomyelia,
diplomyelia, myelatelia, myelocyst,
myelocystocele, myelodysplasia
spinal cord destruction: myelodiastasis
spinal cord dilation: syringomyelus
spinal cord diseases: arachnoiditis,
cauda equina syndrome,
holorachischisis, merorachischisis,
mesorachischisis, myelauxe,
myelopathy, myelosclerosis,
necrobiosis, pneumorrachis,
poliomyelopathy, syringomelia
spinal cord examination: myelography
spinal cord hernia: meningomyelocele,
myelocele, myelomingocele, spina
bifida

spinal cord inflammation: ixomyelitis, myelitis, myelomeningitis, myeloradiculitis, spinal meningitis, syringomyelitis
spinal cord opening: myelopore
spinal cord paralysis: myeloparalysis, myeloplegia
spinal cord softening: myelomalacia
spinal cord surgery: chordotomy, cordotomy, myelorrhaphy, myelotomy
spinal cord tumor: chordoma
spinal cord wasting: myelatrophy
spinal fluid deficiency: anhydromyelia
spine: *See* vertebral column
spindle-shaped: fusiform
spineless: invertebrate
spiny: acantho-, echino-, acanthoid, echinate, spicule
spiral: Curachmann's, helix, volute
spirit: anima, alcohol
spit: expectoration, ptysis, saliva, slaver, spittle, sputum
spit causing: expectorant
spit inducer: sialagogue
splashing sound: capotement
splayfoot: pes planus, talipes valgus
spleen: lien-, lieno-, splen-, spleno-, lien, lienal
spleen, absence: alienia, asplenia
spleen, originating in: splenogenic
spleen, small: microsplenia
spleen bleeding: splenorrhagia
spleen congestion: splenemia, splenemphraxis
spleen disease: autosplenectomy, splenectopia, splenopathy
spleen enlargment: hypersplenism, megalosplenia, splenadenoma, splenectasia, splenomegaly
spleen excision: splenectomy
spleen fixation: exosplenopexy, splenopexy
spleen hardening: splenceratosis, splenoceratosis, splenokeratosis
spleen hernia: lienocele, splenocele

spleen incision: splenotomy
spleen inflammation: episplenitis, lienitis, perisplenitis, splenicterus, splenitis
spleenlike: spleniform, splenoid
spleen pain: splenalgia, splenodynia
spleen prolapse: splenonephroptosis, splenoptosis
spleen softening: lienomalacia, splenomalacia, splenomyelomalacia
spleen suturing: splenorrhaphy
spleen tumors: splenoma, splenoncus
spleen ulceration: splenelcosis
splice: anastomose, graft, interface, juncture
splinter: pulverize
split: schisto-, schizo-, aperture, bifurcate, bisect, channel, cleavage, cleft, dehiscence, divide, fission, furrow, rupture, segmentation
spoil: decompose, deteriorate, putrefy
spongelike: spongiform, spongioid
spongy: cancellous, resilient
spontaneous generation: abiogenesis, heterogenesis
spoon nail: koilonychia
spoon-shaped: cochleariform
spore-forming: sporogenesis
spore-producing: sporiferous
sport: mutation
spot: blemish, blotch, loculus, macula, milium, nevus, papilla, papule, pustule
spout: discharge, duct, eject
spray: atomizer, disseminate
spread: contagion, diffuse, dilation, dispersion, distension, effuse, metastasis, radiate, transmission
spread apart: patulous
spring back: rebound
springy: elasticity, flexibility, resilience
sprinkle: disperse, disseminate, droplet
sprout: bud, develop, germinate, grow
spume: discharge, eject, emit

spur: calcar, lacerate, puncture
spur-shaped: calcarine
spurt: effusion, ejaculation, emission,
    flux, vomit
sputum, albumin in: albuminoptysis
sputum, blood in: hemoptysis
squeeze: compress, constrict, express
squint: cyclotropia, esotropia,
    exotropia, heterotropia, strabismus,
    tropia
S-shaped curve: ogive
stab: band cell, lancinate, prick,
    puncture, trauma, wound
stable: dormant, inert, quiescent
staff: caduceus, cane, crutch
stagger: fluctuation, titubation
stagnation: deterioration, obstruction,
    stasis, topor
staining, double: dichromophilism
staining easily: chromaphile,
    chromatophil
staining poorly: amblychromasia,
    amblychromatic, chromophobia
stains: acid, basic, Cajal's, contrast,
    counterstain, dye, Ehrlich's,
    fluorescent, Giemsa, Golgi's
    Gomori's, Gram's, hematoxylin-
    eosin, Koster, lipid, Loeffler's,
    Machiavello, Masson's trichrome,
    May-Grunwald, metachromatic,
    methylzine blue, neutral, Nissl's,
    Papanicolaou, Pappenheim's,
    periodic acid-Schiff, pigment,
    Sudan, van Gieson's, von Kossa,
    Wright's, Ziehl-Neelsen
stalk: pedicle, peduncle, petiole, pila,
    pillar
stammer: battarismus, dysphemia,
    lingual titubation, paralalia,
    psellism, stutter
stand, inability to: anastasia
standing: orthograde
standing difficulty: amyostasia,
    astasia, dysstasia
standing up, fear of: stasibasiphobia,
    stasiphobia

stapes excision: stapedectomy,
    stapediotenotomy
staphylococci destruction:
    antistaphylococcic
staphylococci in blood:
    staphylococcemia, staphylohemia
starch: amyl-, amylo-, amidin,
    amidulin, amylin, amylogen,
    amylopectin, amylose, amylum
starch, excess in blood: amylemia
starch, excess in feces: amylorrhea
starch, excess in urine: amyluria
starch, inability to digest:
    amylodyspepsia
starch accumulation: amyloidosis
starch conversion: amylolysis
starch eating: amylophagia
starch enzyme: amylase
starch formation: amylogenesis,
    amyloplastic
starch hydrolysis: amylorrhexis
starchlike: amyloid
starch producing: amylogenic
starch synthesis: amylosynthesis
star-shaped: -aster, astro-, asteroid,
    stellate
startle reflex: Moro reflex
starvation: abrosia
state: -acy, -asis, -ecis, -iasis, -osis,
    -sis, condition, status
statistics: biometry, biostatistics
stature, small: microsoma
steal: klepto-
stealing, fear of: kleptophobia
stealing compulsion: kleptomania
steam: atmo-, condensation,
    distillation, vapor
stem: funniculus, habenula, pedicle,
    peduncle, petiole, pila, scapus, stalk
stench: fetid, mephitis, putrescence,
    rancid
stenosis: constriction, obstruction,
    stegnosis
step: ambulation, gait, walk
sterile: antiseptic, asepsis, axenic,
    barren, impotent, infecundity,
    infertility

sterility: acyesis, agenesis
sterilization: hysterectomy, salpingectomy, tubal ligation, vasectomy
sterilize: autoclave
sterum: sterno-, ensisternum, gladiolus, manubrum, plastron, xiphoid process
sternum, absent: asternal
sternum, toward: adsternal
sternum abnormalities: pectus carinatum, pectus excavatum, pectur gallinatum
sternum cleft: sternoschisis
sternum incision: sternotomy
sternum pain: sternalgia, sternodynia
sternum perforation: sternotrypesis
stick: adhere, cane, crutch, glutinous, lancinate, puncture, viscid
stiffness: inflexibility, rigidity, rigor
stiffening, after death: rigor mortis
stiff neck: loxia, torticollis, wryneck
stifle: asphyxiate, choke, repress, suffocate, supress
still: dormant, immobile, inactive, inert, latent, mute, palliate, quiescent, sedate, sedentary, static, tranquilize
stillbirth: fetal death
stimulant: amphetamine, analeptic, antidepressant, caffeine, epinephrine, excitor, neurotransmitter
stimulating: -tropin, pressor, roborant
stimulation: auxo-, horm-, erogenous, excitation, innervation, suscitation
stimulation of adrenal glands: adrenokinetic
stimulation sensitivity: erethism
stimulation threshold: liminal
stimulator: activator
stimulus, low level of: absolute threshold
stimulus, move toward: adient
stimulus avoidance: abient
sting: biotoxin, bite, burn, chafe, irritation, odaxetic

stir: stimulate
stirrup: stapes
stitch: pain, neuralgia, spasm, suturation, suture, tic douloureux, trigeminal neuralgia
stock: funiculus, genotype, genus, peduncle, phenotype, species
stomach: gastro-, cardia, fundus, pyloris, ventriculus
  See also abdomen
stomach, abnormal: ectasia
stomach, absence of: agastria
stomach, enlarged: gastrectasia, gastromegaly, megalogastria
stomach, lying on: prone, ventricumbent
stomach, on right of: dextrogastria
stomach, small: microgastria
stomach, study of: gastrology
stomach, upset: dyspepsia
stomachache: gastralgia, gastrodynia
stomach acid, excess: chlorhydria
stomach acid, test for: Bernstein
stomach bleeding: gastrorrhagia, gastrostaxis
stomach bubble: aerogastria
stomach contents, ejected: emesis, vomit, vomitus
stomach contraction: gastrostenosis
stomach diseases: chalasia, gastromycosis, gastropathy, gastroschisis, gastrosis, ulcer
stomach displacement: gastroptosis
stomach examination: gastroscopy, stomachoscopy
stomach excision: antrectomy, Billroth I, II, cardiectomy, gastrectomy, gastropulorectomy
stomach fistula: gastrostoma
stomach foulness: saburra, sordes
stomach glands, inflammation: gastradenitis
stomach hernia: gastrocele
stomach inflammation: endogastritis, exogastritis, gastritis, gastroduodenitis, gastroenteritis, gastrojejunitis, linitis, perigastritis

stomach opening: pylorus
stomach pain: cardialgia, gastralgia,
   gastrodynia, peratodynia,
   stomachalgia
stomach paralysis: gastroplegia
stomach region: -ventral
stomach spasm: cardiospasm,
   gastrospasm
stomach specialist: gastroenterologist,
   gastrologist
stomach stone: gastrolith
stomach surgery: cardiectomy,
   fundusectomy,
   gastroduodenostomy,
   gastroenterostomy,
   gastrojejunostomy, gastrolysis,
   gastropexy, gastroplasty,
   gastrorrhapy, gastrostomy,
   pyloroplasty
stomach tooth: lower canine
stomach ulcer: gastrohelcosis, peptic
stomach wasting: gastratrophia
stone: lith-, -lith, litho-, petro-,
   calculus, cholelithiasis, concretion,
   gallstone, scybalum, sympexion
stone crushing: lithoclasty,
   lithodialysis, litholapaxy, lithotrity
stone dissolving: lithoclysmia,
   litholysis
stone formation: lithiasis, lithogenesis
stone passage: lithecbole, lithuresis
stone removal: lithectasy, lithocenosis,
   lithogogue, lithotony
stone surgery: lithocystotomy,
   lithonephrectomy, lithotomy
stool: dejecta, excrement, excreta,
   feces, meconium
stools, black: melanorrhagia, melena
stools, fatty: steatorrhea
stools, loose: diarrhea
stoop: hunchback, kyphosis,
   osteoporosis
stop bleeding: hemostasis
stoppage: arrest, blockage, closure,
   compression, constipation,
   embolism, infarct, obstruction,
   remission, stasis

storage: bladder
storage diseases: amaurotic familial
   idiocies, cholesteryl ester,
   gangliosidosis, Gaucher's disease,
   Hunter syndrome, Hurler's
   syndrome, leukodystrophy,
   lipidosis, lipoidosis, mannosidosis,
   Maroteaux-Lamy syndrome,
   Morquio syndrome, mucolipidosis,
   mucopolysaccharidosis, Niemann-
   Pick disease, Sanfilippo syndrome,
   Scheie syndrome, spingolipidosis,
   Tay-Sacks disease, thesaurismosis
storms, fear of: ombrophobia
stout: corpulent, fat, muscular, obese
strabismus: tropia
strabismus surgery: strabotomy
straight: ortho-, recto-, horizontal,
   linear, rectus
straighten: extend, extensor, orthosis,
   rectify
strain: distend, filter, injure, purify,
   separate, sprain
straining: colation
straitjacket: camisole
strand: cilium, fiber, filament, hair,
   ligament
strange: allotrio-, xeno-, aberrant,
   anomalous, atypical, foreign, rare
strangers, fear of: xenophobia
strangle: asphyxiate, constrict,
   obstruct, occlude
strap: band, fascia, ligament, tendon
strapping: healthy, muscular
stratum: lamina, layer, plate
strawberry mark: hemangioma, nevus
   vascularis
streak: band, furrow, linea, stria,
   striation, strip, stripe, variegate,
   vein
stream: effluvium, ejaculation,
   emanation, flux
street crossing, fear of: dromophobia
strength: dynamo-, stheno-, potency,
   reinforcement, resilience,
   resistance, stenia, vitality

strength, lack of: atony
strength, normal: sthenia
strength, reduce: attenuate
strengthening: antasthenic
strength measurement: sthenometry
streptococci destruction:
    antistreptococcic
streptococci in blood: strepticemia,
    streptococcemia
stress: pressure, stimulus, strain,
    tension, test
stress ulcer: Curling's ulcer
stretch: elastic, extension, resilience,
    strain, syntasis
stretcher: gurney, litter
stretching: ectatic, pandiculation,
    parectasia, tension
stretch mark: stria
stricken: injured, wounded
stricture: coarctation, compression,
    constriction, contraction,
    strangulation
stricture cutting: coarctotomy
stride: gait
strident: guttural, hoarse
string: chord-, catgut, fiber, filament,
    ligament, suture, thread
stringy: fibrous, filamentous, glutinous,
    mucilaginous, mucoid
strip: desquamation, ebuviation,
    excoriation, molt, slough
stripe: linea, stratum, striate, striation
stroke: -plegia, apoplexy, brain
    hemorrhage, cerebral thrombosis,
    cerebrovascular accident, coup,
    ictus
stroke, after: postictal
stroke, false: parapoplexy,
    pseudoapoplexy
stroking: effleurage, frottage
strokelike: apoplectiform, apoplectoid
strong: muscular, sthenic, virile
structural support: tenosuspension
structure: form, morphology, physique
structure, accessory: adnexia
structure, study of: anatomy

structure, without: anhistic
structure-function: biostatics
study of: -ology
stumbling: titubation
stun: anesthetize, shock, stupefy
stunt: abort, arrest, dwarf, midget,
    pygmy, restraint
stupefied: anesthetized, comatose,
    drugged, unconscious
stupid: See mental retardation
stupor: narco-, catatonia, comatose,
    narcohypnosis, narcosis,
    psychocoma, sopor
stupor causing: carotic, narcotic,
    soporific, stupefacient
stuttering: anarthria literalis,
    battarismus, lingual titubation,
    psellism, spasmophemia,
    stammering
St. Vitus dance: choria
sty: hordeolum, tarsophyma
styloid process, inflammation:
    styloiditis
subconscious: repressed, subliminal,
    unconscious
subcostal nerve pain: subcostalgia
subdivision: class, family, genus, order,
    phylum, section, segment, species,
    taxon
subdue: abate, palliate, remission,
    restraint, tranquilize
subject: case, expose, index case,
    patient, propositus
submaxillary gland inflammation:
    submaxillaritis, submaxillitis
subnormal: deficient, mentally
    retarded
subside: abate, remission
subsidiary: adjuvant, ancillary,
    auxiliary
subsistence: alimentation,
    maintenance, nutriment
substance: density, marrow, mass,
    matter, medium, viscosity
substance impurity: adulteration
substances, separation of: analysis

substitute: locum tenens,
   succedaneous, surrogate
substrate: zymolyte
succession: proximate, series, sequence
succumb: deteriorate, die, expire
suck in: inhale, respire
sucking: myzesis
suckling: breast feed, lactation
suck out: aspirate
suction: ablation, aspiration
sudden onset: acute
suffering: grief, pain, stress, trauma
suffocate: asphyxiate
suffuse: diffuse, infuse, saturate
sugar: gluco-, saccharo-,
   carbohydrate, dextrose, fructose,
   galactose, glucose, lactose, levulose,
   maltose, saccharum, simple, sucrose
sugar disease: diabetes mellitus
sugar in blood: glucohemia, glycemia,
   gylcosemia, sucrosemia
sugar in blood, decreased:
   hypoglycemia
sugar in blood, increased:
   hyperglycemia, hyperglycoplasmia
sugar in body fluids: saccharorrhea
sugar in cerebral spinal fluid:
   glycorrhachia, hyperglycorrhachia
sugar in tissues, decreased: glycopenia
sugar in urine: glucosuria, glycosuria,
   hyperglycosuria, melituria,
   saccharosuria, saccharuria,
   sucrosuria
suggestibility: sympathism
suggestion: hypnotism, mesmerism,
   pathetism, pithiatism
suitable: compatible, congruent
sulfur: sulfo-, thio-
sulfur in blood, excessive: thiemia
sun: helio-
sunder: dehiscence, dissociation,
   rupture, section, split
sunlight treatment: heliation,
   heliotherapy
sunstroke: coup de soleil, heliosis,
   insolation, siriasis, thermoplegia

superior: super-
superstition: delusion, fanaticism
supplement: accessory, ancillary,
   auxiliary
support: alimentation, bandage, brace,
   corset, crutch, maintenance,
   nutriment, reinforce, sling, splint,
   stent, strap, suspension, sustain,
   sustentacular, trabs, truss
support needs: anaclisis
suppository: turunda
suppression: ischio-, arrest, blockage,
   confinement, obstruction, restraint,
   stoppage
suppuration: discharge, excretion,
   gleet, ichor, leukorrhea, pus, sanies
surface: integument, local, skin,
   stratum, topical
surface attachment: adsorption
surface tension agent: surfactant
surgery: Abbe's, Adams', Ammon's,
   anaplasty, Arlt's, Babcock's,
   Baldy's, Barsky's, Bassini's, Beck,
   Billroth's, Blalock-Taussig,
   bloodless, Bowman's, Brunschwig's,
   Caldwell-Luc, Cecil's, cesarean,
   Charnley, cosmetic, Cushing's,
   Dandy, Dupuy-Dutemps, Elliot's,
   Emmet's, Estes', exploratory,
   extraction, fenestration, flap,
   Freund's, Gilliam's, Gillie's, Gil-
   Vernet, Graefe's, Halstead's,
   Herbert's, Hibbs', Hill, Huggins',
   Hunter's, interval, Kelly's,
   Killian's, Kocher's, Littre,
   McBurney's, major, Matas', Mayo's,
   Mikulicz's, minor, Mustard,
   Naffziger's, neoplasty, neostomy,
   Ober's, Payne's, plastic, Polya's,
   Pomeroy's, Potts, radical, Rastelli's,
   Roux-en-Y, seton, shelf, Smith,
   Syme's, Talma's, Tanner's, TeLinde,
   Trendelenburg, Treves', Urban's,
   Vineberg's, Wagner's, Wertheim's,
   Whipple's, Whitehead's, Young's,
   Ziegler's
   See also individual organs

surgery, after: postoperative
surgery, before: preoperative
surgery, for study: biotomy, vivisection
surgical aid: bandage, bucrylate,
epinephrine, flucrylate, mecrylate,
ocrylate, polybutester, polybutilate,
polydioxanone, polygalactin,
polyglyconate, suture
surgical instruments: agraffe,
Bigelow's lithotrite, bilabe,
bistoury, bougie, catlin, clamp,
clasp, clip, compressor, curet,
dermatome, dilator, director, file,
fleam, forceps, glide, gorget, gouge,
guillotine, hemostat, hook,
hymenotome, kiotome, knife,
labiotenaculum, lancet, lithotrite,
needle, needleholder, operation
microscope, ophthalmostat,
osteoclast, osteotome, osteotrite,
probe, proctotome, protractor,
punch, rangeur, rasp, raspatory,
retractor, saw, scalpel, scalprum,
scarificator, scarifier, scissors,
scoop, separator, separatorium,
septotome, serrefine, serrenoeud,
seton, snare, sound, spatula,
specillum, splanchnotribe, spoon,
spud, staphylotome, stapler, stent,
stilet, stylet, styliscus, stylus,
tenaculum, trephine, trocar,
uvulotome, xyster
surgical joining: anastomosis, bypass
surgical procedures: allongement,
anastomosis, cryosurgery, cutdown,
electrocoagulation, electrosurgery,
laser, photocoagulation
surgical removal: amputation, excision
surrounded: encapsulated, encysted
surrounding: circum-, peri-, ambient
survey: analysis, examination,
investigation, monitor, probe,
research, study
susceptibility: predilection,
predisposition, proneness
suspend: arrest, inactivate

sustain: alimentation, maintenance,
nutrition, support
sutures: -rhaphy, absorbable,
atraumatic, buried, button, catgut,
chain stitch, continuous, figure-
of-eight, flat, guy, ligature,
mattress, nonabsorbable, pterion,
pulley, pursestring, retention,
rhinion, schindylesis, silk, tension,
through and through, wire
suture over: enkatarrhaphy
swab: abstergent, cotton, gauze, scrub,
sponge
swallowing: absorption, assimilation,
deglutition, imbibition, ingestion
swallowing, excessive: sialoaerophagy
swallowing, pain with: odynophagia
swallowing air: aerophagia
swallowing disorder: aglutition,
aphagia, dysphagia
swamp fever: malaria, paludism
sweat: sudo-, excretion, perspiration,
sudor
sweat, blood in: hematidrosis
sweat, blue: cyanephidrosis,
cyanhidrosis
sweat, colored: chromhidrosis,
melanephidrosis
sweat, luminescent: phosphorhidrosis,
phosphoridrosis
sweat, milklike: galactidrosis
sweat, odor of: bromhidrosis,
osmidrosis
sweat, odorous in armpit:
tragomaschalia
sweat, urea in: uridrosis
sweat bath: sauna, sudatorium,
turkish
sweat formation: hidropoiesis, hidrosis,
idrosis, sudoriferous, sudoriparous
sweat gland: apocrine, eccrine
sweat gland diseases: anaphoresis,
miliaria rubra, sudamen,
sudorikeratosis, tropical lichen
sweat gland inflammation:
hidradenitis, hydradenitis

sweat gland treatment:
hydrosudotherapy
sweat gland tumors: hidradenoma,
hidrocystoma, hydradenoma,
spiradenoma, spiroma,
syringadenoma,
syringocystadenoma,
syringocystoma, syringoma
sweating: hidrosis, perspiration,
sudation
sweating, abnormal: hemidiaphoresis,
hemidrosis, hemihidrosis,
hemihyperhydrosis, hidrorrhea,
hidroschesis, hidrosis,
hyperhidrosis, hypohidrosis, idrosis,
paridrosis
sweating, absence of: adiaphoresis,
anhidrosis, anidrosis, hidroschesis,
hypolidrosis
sweating, excessive: desudation,
diaphoresis, ephidrosis,
hyperephidrosis, hyperhidrosis,
polyhyrosis, sudoresis, synidrosis
sweating, in armpit: maschalephidrosis
sweating, normal: eudiaphoresis
sweating, over entire body:
panhidrosis
sweat prevention: anhidrotic,
antihidrotic, antipersperant,
antisudorific, deodorant, ischidrosis
sweat promoting: diaphoretic, sudorific
sweet air: nitrous oxide
sweetening: edulcorant
sweet taste: glycogeusia
swelling: -cele, anasarca, dilation,
distention, edema, enlargement,
glomus, hypertrophy,
intumescence, node, prominence,
protuberance, torus, tuber,
tumescence, tumefaction,
tumentia, tumor, turgescence,
turgid
swelling, air-filled: aerocele
swelling of hand or foot: acroedema
swelling reduction: decongestant,
detumescence

swift: tachi-, tacho-, tachy-
swimmer's itch: schistosome
dermatitis
swing: fluctuate, pendulous, vibrate
swirl: agitate, circulate, rotate
switch: anastomosis, bypass,
divergence, substitute, transpose
swoon: faint, syncope, unconsciousness
sword-shaped: ensiform, xiphoid
symmetrical: actinomorphous,
congruent, isogonal, isomerism,
isomorphous, proportional
sympathetic ganglion pain:
sympatheticalgia
sympathetic nerve disorder:
sympathicolytic, sympathicotonia
sympathetic nerve inflammation:
sympathiconeuritis
sympathetic nerve surgery:
sympathectomy, sympathicectomy
symposium: colloquy, conference,
congress
symptom: disease, indication, sign,
syndrome, trait
symptom improvement: decrudescence,
remission
symptoms, lack of: asymptomatic
symptoms, science of: semeiotics,
semiotics
symptoms, study of: semeiology,
semiology, symptomatology
synchronous: concomitant, concurrent,
isochronia
synovial fluid, lack of: asynovia
synovial inflammation: parasynovitis,
synovitis
synovial joint: ball-and-socket, hinge,
gliding, pivot
synovial membrane excision:
synovectomy
synovial membrane tumor: synovioma
synthesis: admixture, alloy,
amalgamation, fusion, healing,
union
synthetic: artifact, imitation, pseudo,
simulated

syphilis: spirochete
syphilis, diseases from: dementia paralytica, neurosyphilis
syphilis, fear of: syphiliphobia, syphilomania, syphilophobia
syphilis development: syphilogenesis
syphilis disorder: syphilopathy, syphilophyma
syphilis-like: syphiloid
syphilis test: Kahn, VDRL, Wassermann
syphilis therapy: antiluetic, antisyphilitic
syphilis tumor: gumma, syphiloma
syphilis ulcer: syphilelcosis, syphilelcus
system: method, organization, pattern, procedure, process, regimen, schema
systemic feeding: alimentotherapy, parenteral nutrition
systole, before: perisystole, presystole

T

tabes, fear of: tabophobia
tabeslike: tabetiform
table: chart, examination, graph, lamina, operating, plate
tablet: bolus, capsule, lozenge, pill, troche
tacit: aphonia
tactile: *See* touch
tactile sense, blunted: hypopselaphesia
tag: affix, appendage, conjoin, flap, label, projection, protuberance
tail: caud-, appendage, cauda, caudate, flagellum
tailbone: coccyx
tailless: acaudate
tailward: caudad
taint: contagion, contamination, discoloration, infection, macula, poison, pollution, predisposition, stigma
take: absorb, assimilate, drink, eat, ingest, swallow

talk: *See* speech
talkativeness, excessive: hyperphasia, logorrhea, panglossia
tall: gigantism
tamper: adulterate, contaminate, pollute
tangent: convergent, intersect, juxtapose, proximate
tantrum: convulsion, paroxysm, seizure, spasm
tap: decant, drain, percuss, probe, puncture, valve
tapeworm: cestode, Echinococcus, Hymenolepis, Diphyllobothrium, Taenia
tapeworm, against: taeniacide, taeniafuge
tapeworm, fear of: taeniophobia
tapeworm diseases: echinococcosis, hymenolepiasis, hymenolepidosis, taeniasis
tapeworm infestation: cysticercosis, diphyllobathriasis, sparganosis
tapeworm-like: cestoid, taeniform
tarsal excision: tarsectomy
tarsal fracture: tarsoclasia
tarsal inflammation: tarsitis
taste: degustation, gustation, heterogeusia
taste, abnormal: ageusia, dysgeusia, pseudogeusesthesia, pseudogeusia
taste, acute: hypergeusesthesia, hypergeusia, oxygeusia
taste, blunted: amblygeustia, cacogeusia, hemigeusia hypogeusia, parageusia, phantogeusia, pseudogeusia
tattoo removal: dermabrasion
taut: strained, tense
tax: exhaust, fatigue, strain
tea posisoning: theaism
tear: cleft, dehiscence, disintegrate, fissure, lacerate, lacrimal secretion, rupture, wound
tear apart: dilaceration, rupture
tear away: avulsion, evulsion

tear duct: canaliculus
    See also lacrimal duct
tear duct calculus: ophthalmolith
tear duct inflammation: dacryocystitis
tear gland inflammation:
    dacryoadenitis
tearing: dacryops, dacryorrhea,
    delacrimation, epiphora,
    illacrimation
tears: dacry-, dacryo-, lacrimation
tears, abnormal: dacryohemorrhea,
    dacryopyorrhea
tears, absence: alacrima
tears, stimulating: dacryogenic,
    dacryogogue
teat: mammae, nipple, papilla
technique: manner, method,
    methodology, procedure
teenage: adolescent, immature,
    juvenile, pubescent
teeth: dent-, denta-, denti-, dento-,
    odont-, odonto-, canines, incisors,
    molars, premolars
    See also tooth
teeth, absence: anodontia, edentia,
    edentulous
teeth, accumulation: sordes
teeth, cutting: odontiasis
teeth, excessive number: polydontia
teeth, false: denture
teeth, large: macrodontia, megadontia,
    megalodontia
teeth, malaligned: abocclusion
teeth, two sets: diphyodont
teeth grinding: bruxism, bruxomania,
    odontoprisis
teethlike: pectinate, pectiniform
temperament: cerebrotonic, diathesis,
    predisposition, somatotonic,
    viscerotonic
temperance: abstinence, nephalism
temperature: febrile, fever,
    hyperpyrexia, pyrexia
temperature, subnormal: hypothermia
temperature measurement: pyometer,
    thermometer

temperature scale: Celsius, Fahrenheit
temporal bone inflammation: petrositis
temporary: impermanent, temporal,
    transient
tenacious: adhesive, cohesive,
    glutinous, mucilaginous,
    persistence, strength, viscid
tend: doctor, nurse, nurture
tendency: predisposition, tropism
tender: inflamed, irritated, painful,
    pia, sensitive, sore, undeveloped
tendon: tendo-, teno-, chorda
tendon disease: onkinocele,
tendon excision: tenectomy,
    tenonectomy, tenosynovectomy
tendon hardening: tenostosis
tendon incision: tendotomy,
    tenomyotomy, tenotomy
tendon inflammation: tendinitis,
    tendosynovitis, tendovaginitis,
    tenonitis, tenontothecitis, tenositis,
    tenosynovitis, tenovaginitis,
    thecitis
tendon pain: teinodynia, tenalgia,
    tenodynia, tenontodynia
tendon surgery: tendinoplasty,
    tendolysis, tendoplasty, tenolysis,
    tenomyoplasty, tenontomyoplasty,
    tenontomyotomy, tenontoplasty,
    tenoplasty
tendon suturing: tendinosuture,
    tenorrhaphy, tenosuture
tendon tumor: desmoid
tennis elbow: epicondylitis
tension: tonic
tension, abnormal: hypertonia
tension, uniform: homotonic
tenth cranial nerve: vagus
termination: telo-
terminology: nomenclature,
    onomatology
terms: menstruation
terror: enosimania, fear, fright
testes: orchido-, orchis, testicle
testes, abnormal: monorchial,
    monorchism, parorchidium,
    polyorchidism, synorchism,
    triorchidism

testes, absent: agenosomia, anorchism
testes, dropped: orchidoptosis
testes, undescended: cryptorchidism,
    cryptorchism
testes disease: orchiopathy
testes excision: castration,
    cryptorchidectomy, gonadectomy,
    orchiectomy, testectomy
testes fusion: synorchism
testes hardening: orchioscirrhus
testes incision: orchiotomy
testes inflammation: didymitis,
    orchiepididymitis, orchitis,
    pachyvaginalitis, periorchitis,
    testitis
testes membrane: albuginea testis
testes pain: didymalgia, orchialgia,
    orchiodynia, orchioneuralgia
testes spasm: orchichorea
testes surgery: orcheoplasty,
    orchidopexy, orchiodotomy,
    orchiopexy, orchioplasty,
    orchiorrhapy
testes swelling: hydrocele
testes tumors: androblastoma,
    orchidoncus, orchiocele, orchioncus,
    sarcocele, seminoma, Sertoli cell
    tumor
testosterone derivative: anabolic
    steroid
tests: acetone, achievement, Adson's,
    agglutination. albumin, Allen's,
    Almer's, alpha, Amann's, Ames,
    aminopyrine, Amsler, analysis,
    angiocardiography, angiography,
    apperception, aptitude, Aschheim-
    Zondek, assay, association, Ayer's,
    Becker's, Bènder gestalt,
    Benedict's, benzidine, Bernstein,
    beta, Bing, biopsy, Borden's,
    bromsulphalein, bronchoscopy,
    caloric, centesis, chi-square,
    cineangiocardiography,
    coagulation, Cohn's, computed
    tomography, Coomb's, creatine,
    dextrose, Dick, Doppler
    cardiography, Dugas,
    echoencephalography,
    electrocardiography,
electroencephalography, Emmens',
endoscopy, estrogen-receptor
assay, ether, evoked potentials,
examination, exploratory,
fetoscopy, flocculation, fluorescent
antibody test, fluoroscopy, foam,
fragility, Frei, gel diffusion, glucose
tolerance, guaiac, Guthrie, Ham,
histamine, Howard, hue, indole,
intelligence, investigation, Janet's,
Jolles', Kahn, kidney function,
Kveim-Siltzbach, Lange's, latex
agglutination, limulus, liver
function, lumbar puncture,
manometry, Mantoux, Marsh's,
Minnesota Multiphasic Personality
Inventory, neutralization, niacin,
nitroblue tetrazolium, nuclear
magnetic imaging, occult blood,
Ouchterlony, Papanicolaou, patch,
personality, phosphatase, platelet
aggregation,
pneumoencephalography,
pregnancy, probe, projective,
prothrombin, provocative,
psychological, psychomotor, Quick's,
Quinlan's, radioallergosorbent,
radiodiagnosis, radiography,
radionuclear scanning, Romberg,
Rorschach, rose bengal, Schick,
Schiller's, Schilling, scratch, skin,
Snellen's, sonography, spot,
Stanford-Binet, stress, subdural
tap, sweat, thematic, tryptophan,
tuberculin, Tzanck, van den
Bergh's, Van Slyke, VDRL,
ventricular puncture,
ventriculography, Wada,
Wassermann
tetanus causing: tetanigenous,
    tetanization
tetanus-like: tetaniform, tetanism,
    tetanoid
tetany test: Trousseau's sign
thalamus: paleothalamus
theory: concept, hypothesis, postulate,
    science, thesis

therapeutic: curative, healing,
   medical, medicinal, recuperative,
   sanatory, surgery
therapies: ablative, acupuncture,
   adjuvant, aerohydrotherapy,
   aerotherapy, aerothermotherapy,
   alkalitherapy, ammotherapy,
   apiotherapy, arsenotherapy,
   aurotherapy, autoanalysis,
   chrysotherapy, clinatotherapy,
   corrective, counterirritation,
   dietotherapy, endocrinotherapy,
   glandular, gold therapy,
   gonadotherapy, group,
   hydrotherapy, hypnotherapy,
   kinesiatrics, massotherapy, music,
   occupational therapy,
   oleochrysotherapy, oleotherapy,
   oleothorax, oxygen,
   pancreatotherapy, physical
   therapy, plasmatherapy,
   psammotherapy, radiation,
   radiotherapy, seismotherapy,
   serotherapy, shock, sitotherapy,
   zomotherapy
therapy, self: autohemotherapy,
   autohypnosis, autoplasmotherapy,
   autoserotherapy, autotherapy,
   autotransfusion
thiamine deficiency disease: beriberi
thick: pach-, pachy-, pycno-, pykno-,
   coagulated, congealed, dense,
   glutinous, sediment, viscid
thicken: inspissate, pyknosis, spissate
thich-skinned: callous, obdurate,
   pachydermatous
thief: kleptomaniac
thigh, between: interfemoral
thigh bone: femur
thigh muscle: adductors, gracilis,
   pectineus, sartorius
thinking: analytic, cerebral, cognitive,
   ratiocinative, rational, reasoning
thinking, illogical: dyslogia
thin: lepto-, attenuation, cachectic,
   emaciated, gaunt

thinness: tenuity
thin physique: ectomorph
third cranial nerve: oculomotor
thirst: dipsesis
thirst, excessive: anadipsia, dipsosis,
   polydipsia
thirst, lack of: adipsia, aposia,
   dehydration, desiccated, oligodipsia
thirst inducer: dipsogen
thoracic duct rupture: chylothorax
thoracic wall inflammation:
   parapleuritis
thorax: pectus
thorax, narrow: stenothorax
thorax fissure: schistothorax
thorax incision: thoracotomy,
   transthoracotomy,
thorn-shaped: spinate
thorny: acantho-, setaceous,
   setiferous, spicular
thoughts, inability to express:
   acataphasia
thread: mito-, catgut, fiber, fibril,
   filament, suture
threadlike: nemato-, fibrillar, fibrous,
   filum, nematoid, piliform
thread-shaped: filiform
three-dimensional: stereo-
three-headed: tricipital
three-pronged: trident
threshold: aperture, entrance, limen
thrill: palpitation, pulsation, vibration
throat: fauces, guttur, jugulum, neck,
   pharynx
throat inflammation: isthmitis,
   laryngitis, sphagitis
throat rattle: rhonchus
throat spasm: gutturotetany,
   laryngospasm
throb: beat, palmus, palpitation,
   pulsate, pulsation
throe: convulsion, ictus, paroxysm,
   spasm, stroke
thrombin, abnormal:
   hyperthrombinemia,
   hypothrombinemia

thrombin deficiency: athrombia
thrombus affinity: thrombophilia
thrombus dissolving: thromboclasis,
thrombocytolysis, thrombolysis
thrombus formation: thrombogenesis
throttle: asphyxiate, compress,
obstruct, occlude, strangulate
through: dia-, per-, trans-
throwback: atavism
throw up: eject, regurgitate, vomit
thrush: candidiasis, candidosis,
moniliasis, mycotic stomatitis
thrust: -tuse, pierce, propel
thumb: pollex
thumb spasm: anticheirotonus
thump: beat, palpitate, pulsate,
vibrate
thunder, fear of: brontophobia
thymus gland: thymo-
thymus gland, abnormal: cacothymia
thymus gland, absence: athymia
thymus gland enlargement:
thymokesis
thymus gland excision: thymectomy,
thymusectomy
thymus gland fixation: exothymopexy,
thymopexy
thymus gland inflammation: thymitis
thymus gland tissue destruction:
thymolysis
thymus gland tumor: thymoma
thymus gland ulceration: thymelcosis
thyroid cartilage incision:
thyrochondrotomy
thyroid gland: thyreo-, thyro-
thyroid gland, absence: athyria,
athyroidism
thyroid gland, normal: euthyroid
thyroid gland, originating in:
thyreogenic
thyroid gland, overactive:
hyperthyroidism, Graves' disease
thyroid gland, underactive: athyreosis,
cretinism, Gull's disease,
hypothyroidism, myxedema
thyroid gland diseases: dysthyreosis,
dysthyroidism, thyreoprivia,
thyropathy, thyrosis, thyrotoxicosis

thyroid gland enlargment: goiter,
struma, thyrocele
thyroid gland excision: thyroidectomy
thyroid gland fixation: endothyropexy,
exothyropexy
thyroid gland incision: thyroidotomy
thyroid gland inhibitor: antithyroid
thyroid gland inflammation: De
Quervain's thyroiditis, strumitis,
thyroadenitis, thyroiditis
thyroid gland prolapse: thyroptosis
thyroid gland removal: thyroidara,
thyroidectomy
thyroid gland surgery: thyrotomy
thyroid hormone, absence:
athyroidemia
thyroid tissue destruction: thyrolytic
tibia: cnemis, shin
tibia inflammation: cnmitis
tibia pain: tibialgia
tic: neuralgia, spasm, tic douloureux,
twitch
tick: beat, palpitate, pulsate, Ixodes
tick fever: Lyme arthritis, Rocky
Mountain spotted fever, tularemia
tickling sensation: knismogenic,
titillation
tie: bandage, clamp, confine, ligature,
restrain, suture
tight: compressed, constricted,
impermeable, rigid, strained, taut,
tense
tightening: compression, contraction
tilt backward: retroversion
time: chron-, -chronia, chrono-,
duration
time disorder: desynchronosis,
dyschronism, jet lag
tincture: drug, infusion, injection,
medicine, preparation, solution
tine: cusp, projection, spicule
tingle: itch, paresthesia, prickle,
tremor
tip: apex, crown, cusp, head, vertex
tip backward: retroversion
tip forward: anteversion

tiredness: exhaustion, fatigue, lethargy

tissue: histo-, material, matter, substance, substantia, textus

tissue, abnormal development: alloplasia, dysplasia, heteroplasia, heterotopia

tissue, absence: aplasia

tissue, between: interstitial

tissue, dead: gangrene, infarct, mortification, necrosis, radionecrosis, slough, sphacelus

tissue, defective development: hypoplasia

tissue, gas in: aerosis

tissue, overactive: hypermetaplasia

tissue, produced by: histogenous

tissue, spongy: pulp

tissue, study of: histology

tissue, type of: connective, epithelial, muscle, nerve

tissue, urine in: urecchysis, uredema

tissue, white fibrous: albuginea, tunica albuginea

tissue affinity: histaffine

tissue atrophy: cataplasia

tissue cells: histiocyte, histoblast

tissue change: caseation, tyromatosis

tissue contraction: astringent, stypsis

tissue deposit: tophus

tissue destruction: byssocausis, caustic, cauterization, cautery, chemicocautery, chemosurgery, cryocautery, decay, electrocautery, electrodesiccation, electosurgery, escharotic, fulguration, galvanocautery, histodialysis, histolysis, microtomy, moxibustion, photocoagulation, ustion

tissue dissection: histotomy

tissue examination: biospectroscopy, microscopy

tissue excision: biopsy, conization

tissue formation: histogenesis, homeoplasia, protoplasia

tissue hardening: sclerogenous

tissue layer: membrane, panniculus

tissue overproduction: hypergenesis, hyperplasia

tissue removal: debridement, slough

tissue replacement: homoplasty, transubstantiation

tissue response: inflammation

tissue separation: dehiscence, dissection, exfoliation, sloughing

tissue softening: ramollissement

tissue softness: malacosarcosis

tissue transfer: allograft, autograft, explant, graft, heterograft, implant, transplant

tissue tumor: histiocytoma, histoma

toadskin: phrynoderma

tobacco: nicotine, tars

tobacco poisoning: nicotinism, tabacism, tabacosis, tabagism

toe: See digit, extremity, finger, phalanges

toe, large: hallux

toenail: See nail

together: co-. con-, sym-, syn-, concomitant, confluent, conjoined

tone: elasticity, resilience, tension

tone, abnormal: hypertonic, hypotonic

tone, lack of: atony

tone deaf: amusia

tongue: gloss-, glosso-, linguo-, glossa, lingua

tongue, abnormal: ankyloglossia, ateloglossia, glossoptosis

tongue, absent: aglossia, aglossostomia

tongue, beneath: hypoglossal, subglossal, sublingual

tongue, black hairy: glossophytia, melanotrichia lingua

tongue, burning sensation: glossopyrosis

tongue, double: diglossia

tongue, hairy: trichoglossia

tongue, large: macroglossia, megaloglossia

tongue, small: microglossia

tongue, study of: glossology, glottology

tongue biting: odaxesmus
tongue cleft: schistoglossia
tongue discoloration: melapoplakia
tongue diseases: glossopathy, glossophylia, glossoptosis, glossopyrosis
tongue excision: elinguation, glossectomy
tongue incision: glossotomy
tongue inflammation: glossitis, glottitis, paraglossia, paraglossitis, subglossitis
tonguelike: lingula
tongue pain: glossalgia, glossodynia, Moeller's glossitis
tongue paralysis: glossolysis, glossoplegia
tongue surgery: frenotomy, glossoplasty
tongue-tie: ankyloglossia, frenulum linguae
tongue tip: proglossis
tongue tumors: hydroglossia, ranula
tonic: analeptic, medicine, restorative, roborant, stimulant
tonsil abscess: peritonsillar abscess, quinsy
tonsil calculus: amygdalolith, tonsillolith
tonsil diseases: amygdalopathy, tonsillitis, ulceromembranous
tonsil examination: tonsilloscopy
tonsil incision: tonsillotomy
tonsil inflammation: periamygdalitis, peritonsillitis, tonsillitis
tonsil removal: tonsillectomy
tools: See instruments, surgical instruments
tooth: dent-, denta-, denti-, dento-, odont-, odonto-, canine, cuspid, dens, incisor, molar
See also teeth
tooth, absent: agomphiasis, anodontia
tooth, around: peridontal
tooth, artificial: denture, plate, pontic
tooth, broken: odontoclasis

tooth, eye: canine
tooth, fear of: odontophobia
tooth, hard: sclerotic
tooth, milk: deciduous
tooth, permanent: dens permanens
tooth, stomach: lower canine
tooth, wearing away: odontotripsis
toothache: aerodontalgia, dentalgia, odontagra, odontalgia, odontis, odontodynia
toothache reliever: antiodontalgic
tooth calculus: tartar, tophus
tooth cleaner: dentifrice, toothpaste
tooth covering: enamel
tooth cutting: odontiasis
tooth decay: caries, odontonecrosis, saprodontia
tooth decay preventive: anticarious
tooth development: odontogeny
tooth discoloration: amelogenesis imperfecta, xanthodontous
tooth diseases: cavity, cementoma, odontopathy, periodontoclasia, perirhizoclasia
tooth defect: odontatrophy, oligodontia
toothed: dentate, serrate
tooth enamel: adamantine
tooth enamel cell: ameloblast
tooth enamel formation: amelogenesis
tooth erosion: odontotripsis
tooth eruption: odontosis
tooth extraction: exodontia
tooth fissure: odontoschism
tooth formation: odontosis
tooth impression: odontoscopy
tooth incision: odontotomy
tooth inflammation: dentoalveolitis, odontitis, odontobothritis, parodontitis, periodontitis, pyorrhea
toothless: edentulous
toothlike: dentiform, dentoid, odontoid
tooth looseness: odontoseisis
tooth membrane: gingiva

tooth missing: oligodontia
tooth pulled: extraction, odontectomy
tooth root removal: radectomy
tooth socket: odontobothrion
tooth socket bleeding: odontorrhagia,
  phatnorrhagia
tooth socket destruction: alveoloclasia
tooth straightening: orthodontia,
  orthodontics
tooth tissue: dentin
tooth treatment: odontotherapy
tooth tumor: dentinoma,
  dentinosteoid, odontoma
top: acro-, acme, apex, apogee, corona,
  crest, fastigium, vertex
top-shaped: turbinated
torpid: dormant, inanimate, latent,
  lethargic, passive
tortuous: varico-, convoluted, sinuous,
  torsive, varix, volvulate
touch: -aphia, -haphia, hapt-, hapte-,
  hapto-, adjoining, contrectation,
  convergent, intersecting,
  juxtapose, manipulate, massage,
  palpate, pselaphesia, stereognosis,
  tactus, tangent
touched, fear of being: aphephobia,
  haphephobia
touch recognition: symbolia, tactile
touch sense: pselaphesia, stereognosis
touch sense, abnormal: allesthesia,
  allochesthesia, amblyaphia,
  dysaphia, hyperaphia, hypesthesia,
  hypoesthesia, hypopselaphesia,
  paraphia, parapsia, polyesthesia,
  topoanesthesia
touch sense, loss: anaphia,
  apselaphesia, astereognosis,
  stereoagnosis, stereoanesthesia
touch sense, science of: haptics
touch sensitivity: tenderness,
  thigmesthesia, topesthesia,
  topognosia
tourniquet: garrot
toward: ad-, -ad, afferent
toxic: contagious, lethal, morbific,
  pernicious, sapremia, septicemia,
  virulent

toxins: anatoxin, bacteriotoxin,
  biotoxin, choleragen, colitoxin,
  cytolysin, cytost, cytotoxin,
  diphtherin, diphtherotoxin,
  endotoxin, erysipelotoxin,
  erythrotoxin, exotoxin, hemotoxin,
  hepatotoxin, leukociden,
  necrocytotoxin, nephrotoxin,
  neurolysin, neurotoxin, picrotoxin,
  pneumotoxin, poison, tetanolysin,
  toxoid
toxin, acting against: anagotoxic
toxin producing: toxicogenic
toxin removal: detoxification
trace: indication, sign, symptom,
  vestige
trachea: tracheo-
trachea bleeding: tracheorrhagia
trachea dilation: tracheaectasy
trachea disease: tracheopathy
trachea examination:
  tracheobronchoscopy,
  tracheophony, tracheoscopy
trachea fissure: tracheoschisis
trachea hernia: tracheoaerocele,
  tracheocele
trachea incision: tracheolaryngotomy,
  tracheotomy
trachea inflammation: endotracheitis,
  tracheitis, tracheopyosis, trachitis
trachea narrowing: tracheostenosis
trachea pain: trachealgia
trachea softening: tracheomalacia
trachea surgery: tracheoplasty,
  tracheostomy
trains, fear of: siderodromophobia
trance state: catalepsy, coma, hypnotic,
  sopor, stupor
tranquilizers: acetophenozine maleate,
  ataraxic, bromazepam, buspirone,
  chlordiazepoxide, clazolam,
  clobazam, clorazepate, demoxepam,
  gepirone, hydroxyphenamate,
  hydroxyzine, ketazolam, lorzafone,
  loxapine, medazepam, nabilone,
  narcotics, nisobamate, opiates,
  oxazepam, pirenperone, ripazepam,
  rolipram, sedative, sulazepam,

taclamine, temazepam,
triflubazam, tybamate,
valnoctamide
transferable: communicable,
contagious, infectious,
transmissible
transfix: perforate, pierce, puncture
transformation: meta-, conversion,
evolution, halmatogenesis,
metamorphosis, mutation,
permutation, transmutation
transient: evanescent, labile, mutable,
unstable, volatile
transillumination: diaphanoscopy
translucent: hyaline, pellucid,
porcelaneous
transmission: -phoresis, dissimination
transmit disease: communicable,
contagion, infect
transparent: hyaline, pellucid
transplant: allograft, autograft, graft,
heterograft, homograft
transvestism: eonism
trauma: traumato-, injury, lesion,
shock, wound
traveler's diarrhea: giardiasis
traveling, fear of: hodophobia
travel medicine: empariatrics
travel medicine, study of:
hodoiporiatrics
treatment: doctoring, hospitalization,
medication, nursing, surgery,
therapeutics, therapy
treatment, increasing doses:
anatherapeusis
treatment, inhalation of gas:
anapnotherapy
treatment caused: iatrogenic
treatment system: allopathy,
homeopathy
treelike: dendriform, dendritic,
dendroid, ramose
trembling: convulsion, palpitant,
pulsation, tremor, vibration
trembling, fear of: tremophobia
tremor: asterixis, convulsion, fremitus,
jactitation, palpitation, paroxysm,
pulsation, seizure, spasm, subsultus,
synclonus

trench: channel, duct, fossa, furrow,
groove, sulcus
trench mouth: necrotizing gingivitis,
Vincent's angina
trigeminal nerve pain: prosopalgia,
prosopodynia, prosoponeuralgia, tic
douloureux, trigeminal neuralgia
trophoblast: chorion, cytotrophoblast,
placenta, syntrophoblast '
tropical sore: cutáneous leishmaniasis
trough: alve-, canal, channel,
depression, duct, furrow
trunk: torso
trunk, absent: acormus
truth serum: amobarbital
trypanosome destroyer: trypanocide,
trypanosomide
tube: salpingo-, artery, bronchiole,
bronchus, cannula, catheter,
channel, conduit, duct, esophagus,
fallopian, Miller-Abbott, pipette,
salpinx, trachea, vein
tube, dilated: ampulla
tube feeding: gavage feeding,
nasogastric feeding
tubelike: fistulous, syringoid
tuberculosis: phthisis, scrofula
tuberculosis-like: tuberculoid
tuberculosis of spine: Pott's disease,
tuberculous spondylitis
tuberculosis tests: Heaf, Mantoux,
tine, Vollmen patch, von Pirquet
tuberculosis therapy: antituberculotic,
isoniazid, rifampin, tuberculostatic
tuberculosis vaccine: Calmette-Guerin
bacillus
tube removal: extubation
tummy: abdomen, stomach
tummy tuck: abdomenoplasty
tumor, pressure from: oncothlipsis
tumor, study of: oncology
tumor cells, affinity for: oncotropic,
tumoraffin
tumor destruction: oncolysis,
tumoricidal
tumorlike: phymatoid

tumor production: carcinogenesis, oncogenesis, sarcomagenesis, tumorigenesis

tumors: carcino-, cel-, -cele, celo-, -oma, onco-, acanthoma, basiloma, benign, blastoma, bidermoma, branchioma, carcinoma, carcinosarcoma, ceroma, chemodectoma, chloroma, collonema, cylindroma, cystofibroma, cystoma, dermoid cyst, desmocytoma, embryoma, enchonodrosarcoma, endothelioma, epidermoid, epithelioma, Ewing's sarcoma, fibroblastoma, fibroma, ganglioneuroma, hibernoma, leiomyoma, lipofibroma, lymphocytoma, malignant, melanoma, mesothelioma, myeloblastoma, neoplasm, odontoblastoma, odontoma, polyp, sarcoid, sarcoma, telangioma, teratoma, teratocarcinoma
See also individual organs

tumor surgery: lumpectomy, oncotomy

tuning fork: diapason

turbinated bone excision: turbinectomy

turbinated bone incision: turbinotomy

turn: -verse, convolution, intussusception, invagination

turn around: -volute, inversion

turn away: -tropism

turn back: retroflex, retrogression, retroversion

turning: -phoria, anfractuous

turning point: crisis

turn inside out: eversion, exstrophy, introversion, inversion

turn inward: egocentric, enstrophe, idiotropia, inflection, introspective, varus

turn outward: ectropion, eversion

turn upward: supraduction, sursumduction, sursumvergence

twelfth cranial nerve: hypoglossal

twice: bi-, bis-, di-

twinge: cramp, pain, spasm, throb, tic

twins: biovular, conjoined, didymus, dizygotic, fraternal, identical, interlocked, monozygotic, rachiopagus, Siamese, unequal

twins, conjoined: allantoidoangiopagus, anadidymus, anakatadidymus, atlantodidymus, atlodidymus, autosite, cephalodidymus, cephalodiprosopus, cephalopagus, cephalothoracopagus, craniodidymus, craniopagus, cryptodidymus, cyclencephaly, derodidymus, diplopagus, diplosomatia, diprosopus, disomus, duplicitas, ectopagus, epicomus, miopus, omphaloangiopagus, opodidymus, palatopagus, spondylodymus, synadelphus, treophthalmos, tripodia

twisted: strepto-, varico-, valgus

twitch: pulsation, spasm, subsultus, tic, tremor

twitching: ballism, chorea, hemiballism, hemichorea, kymatism, myokymia, synclonus, vellication

two: bi-, bis-, di-, binary, bifurcation, geminate

two-headed: ancipital, dicephaly

two sides: amb-, ambi-, bilateral

tying: ligation

tympanic cavity inflammation: antrotympanitis

type: typo-, category, classification, specimen

type conformity: -typia

typhoid destroyer: typholysin

typhoid fever test: Widal's reaction

typhoid-like: typhoidal

tyrosine in urine: tyrosinuria

tyrosine in urine, excessive: tyrosinosis

U

ulcer: abscess, cancrum, chancre, duodenal, ectrimma, excoriation, furuncle, helcoma, parulis, peptic, phagedena, pustule

ulcer, study of: helcology

ulceration: -angina, aphtha, erosion, gangosa, gangrenous, helicosis, necrotic, septic, sphacelate, suppuration, vomicose

ulcer graft: dermatoplasty

ulcerlike: helcoid

ulcer therapy: cimetidine, doxepin, etintidine, famotidine, metiamide, oxmetidine, ranitidine, sucralfate, tiotidine, trimipramine, zaltidine

ultraviolet radiation, resistant to: uvioresistant

ultraviolet radiation, sensitive to: uviosensitive

umbilical cord: funiculus

umbilicus: omphalo-

umbilicus tumor: sarcomphalocele

unchanging: homeo-, homoco-, homoio-, homeostasis

uncommon: aberrant, anomalous, atypical

unconscious: anesthetic, apsychia, blackout, coma, fainting, id, insensible, narcosis, narcotism, subliminal, syncope

unconsciousness: Adams-Stokes syndrome, petite mal

unconsciousness induction: prenarcosis

uncover: disinterment, exhume, expose

under: cata-, hypo-, infra-, sub-, anesthetized, comatose, hypnotized, unconscious

undernourished: emaciated

understand, inability to: acatalepsia

understanding: cognition, intelligence, perception

understanding, lack of: akatamathesia

undertaker: mortician

undeveloped: immature, rudimentary, vestigial

undivided: ameristic

undulant fever: brucellosis, melitensis

unequal: aniso-, amorphous, asymmetric, disproportional

uneven: anomalo-

unfermented: azymic

unguent: abirritant, balm, demulcent, embrocation, emollient, liniment, ointment, salve

unhealthy: enervated, insalubrious, morbific, peccant, septic, toxic, valetudinarian, virulent

uniform: analogous, equivalent, homogenous, symmetric

union: co-, con-, zygo-, amalgamate, articulation, coalesce, confluence, convergence, fusion, graft, hybrid, junction, linkage, mosaic, synthesis

unknown, fear of: neophobia

unknown cause: cryptogenic, idiopathic

unlike: atypical, heterogeneous, variant

unnatural: aberrant, abnormal, anomalous, monster, nonviable, perverse, teras

unpaired: azygous, impar

unprotected: exposed, nonimmune, pregnable, susceptible, unvaccinated, vulnerable

unreality, feelings of: depersonalization

unresponsive: frigidity, refractory

unsanitary: contaminated, impure, insalubrious, morbific, noxious, polluted, septic, toxic, unhygienic

unsex: castrate, emasculate

unsound: anemic, cachetic, diseased, ill, infected, infirm, mentally ill, mentally retarded, unhealthy, valetudinarian

unstable: fluctuation, labile, mutable, volatile

unsteady gait: ataxia
uphold: sustentacular
upon: ep-, epi-
uptake: absorption, assimilation
upright: orthostatic
upward: an-, ana-
urachus, pus in: pyourachus
urea, reduced: hypoazoturia
urea formation: ureagenesis
urea in blood, excessive: azotemia,
   uremia
urea in sweat: urhidrosis, uridrosis
ureter, bleeding: ureterorrhagia
ureter, enlarged: megaloureter
ureter, mucus in: ureterophlegma
ureter, pus in: pyoureter
ureter calculus: ureterolith
ureter calculus development:
   ureterolithiasis
ureter dilation: ureterectasis,
   ureterohydronephrosis
ureter disease: ureteropathy
ureter examination:
   chromoureteroscopy, ureterography
ureter excision: ureterectomy,
   ureteronephrectomy
ureter incision: ureterolithotomy,
   urethrotomy, uroterotomy
ureter inflammation: ureteritis,
   ureteropyelitis,
   ureteropyelonephritis,
   ureteropyosis
ureter narrowing: ureterostenosis
ureter pain: ureteralgia
ureter prolapse: ureterocele
ureter rupture: ureterodialysis,
   ureterolysis
ureter surgery: ureterocolostomy,
   ureteroenterostomy,
   ureteroneocystostomy,
   ureteroneopyelostomy,
   ureteroplasty, ureteroproctostomy,
   ureterorectoneostomy,
   ureterosigmoidostomy,
   ureterostomy,
   ureteroureterostomy,
   ureterovesicostomy

ureter suture: ureterorrhaphy
urethra: urethro-
urethra abnormality: anaspadias,
   ankylurethria, epispadias,
   hypospadias, paraspadias
urethra bleeding: urethrorrhagia,
   urethrostaxis
urethra discharge: gleet, urethrorrhea
urethra examination:
   aerourethroscopy, urethrography,
   urethroscopy
urethra excision: urethrectomy
urethra fixation: urethropexy
urethra hernia: urethrocele
urethra incision: urethrotomy
urethra inflammation: bulbitis,
   preurethritis, urethritis,
   urethrocystitis
urethra narrowing: urethrostenosis
urethra obstruction: urethratresia,
   urethremphraxis, urethrophraxis
urethra pain: urethralgia
urethra spasm: urethrism,
   urethrospasm
urethra surgery: meatotomy,
   stricturotomy, urethroplasty,
   urethrostomy
urethra suturing: urethrorrhaphy
urethra tumor: urethrophyma
urge: drive, force, impulse, motivation,
   stimulus, stress
urgent: critical, emergency, severe,
   stat
uric acid: urico-
uric acid decomposition: uricolysis
uric acid deficiency in blood:
   hypourocemia
uric acid deficiency in urine:
   hypouricuria
uric acid in bile: uricocholia
uric acid in blood, excessive:
   hyperuricemia, uricacidemia,
   uricemia
uric acid in urine, excessive:
   hyperuricuria, lithuria,
   uricaciduria, uricosuria

uric acid production: uricopoiesis
urinary tract disease: uropathy
urinary tract ulceration: urelcosis
urination: micturition, uresis
urination, abnormal: chaude-pisse,
    opsiuria, paruria, strangury,
    uracrasia
urination, decreased: hypourocrinia,
    oliguria, uropenia
urination, drug for: diuretic
urination, excessive: hydruria,
    hyperdiruesis, nocturia, nycturia,
    pollakiuria, polyuria, thamuria
urination, involuntary: enuresis,
    incontinent, uracratia, uroclepsia,
    urorrhea
urination, normal: orthuria
urination, normal inclination:
    uresiesthesia, uriesthesis
urination, painful: dysuria, urodynia
urination, slow: bradyuria
urination difficulty: acraturesis,
    anuria, dysuria, oligakisuria,
    tenesmus
urination inducer: diuretic, uragogue
urine: uro- urono-, egesta
urine, in: -uria
urine, abnormal: allotriuria
urine, abnormal color: chromaturia,
    melanuria, urocyanosis
urine, absence of bile in: acholuria
urine, acid in: aciduria
urine, albumin in: albuminaturia,
    albuminorrhea, albuminuria
urine, alcohol in: alcoholuria
urine, alkali in: alkalinuria, alkaluria
urine, amebae in: ameburia
urine, amines in, excessive:
    aminosuria, aminuria
urine, amino acids in, excessive:
    aminoaciduria
urine, ammonia in, excessive:
    ammoniuria
urine, amylase in, excessive:
    amylasuria
urine, blood in: hematuria

urine, calculus in: urocheras, urolith,
    uropsammus
urine, chlorides in, excessive:
    chloriduria
urine, cloudiness of: nebula, nubecula
urine, colorless: achromaturia,
    albiduria, albinuria
urine, dark: alkaptonuria
urine, decreased secretion: oliguria
urine, excess water in: polyhydruria
urine, gas in: pneumatinuria,
    pneumaturia, pneumouria
urine, hemoglobin in: hemoglobinuria
urine, increased pH: alkalinuria,
    alkaluria
urine, milky: chyluria, galacturia
urine, porphyrin in: porphyrinuria,
    porphyuria
urine, pus in: pyuria
urine, red: erythuria
urine, spicy odor: uraroma
urine concentration, high:
    oligohydruria
urine concentration, low: hydruria
urine containing: urinose
urine diagnosis: uromancy
urine formation: uropoiesis
urine in cyst: urinoma, uroncus
urine in feces: urochezia
urine in tissues: urecchysis, uredema,
    uroedema
urine poisoning: urosepsis, urotoxicity
urine producing: uriniparous,
    urinogenous, urogenous
urine retention: anuresis, anuria
urine secretion reducer: antidiuretic
urine secretor: nephron
urine suppression: ischuria, uroschesis
urobilin in blood: urobilinemia
urobilin in urine, excessive:
    urobilinuria
urobilinogen in blood:
    urobilinogenemia
usual: normo-, habitual, standard
utensil: apparatus, instrument, vessel
uterus: hystero-, metra-, metro-,
    womb

uterus, abnormal: anteflexion, anteversion, retroflexion, retroversion

uterus, absence: ametria

uterus, blood in: hematometra

uterus, double: didelphia, dihysteria, dimetria

uterus, dropped: hysteroptosia, metroptosis, procidentia, prolapsed, proptosis

uterus, lack of: ametria

uterus, narrow: metrostenosis

uterus, near: parametrial

uterus, outside of: ectopic, extrauterine

uterus, reduced: hyperinvolution, superinvolution

uterus, softening: metromalacia, metromalacosis

uterus atrophy: metratrophia

uterus bleeding: metrorrhagia, metrostaxis

uterus calculus: hysterolith, uterolith

uterus contractions: Ahlfeld's sign

uterus cyst formation: metrocystosis

uterus descent into pelvis: lightening

uterus dilation: lochiometra, metrectasia

uterus discharge: lochia, metrorrhea

uterus diseases: Asherman syndrome, hematometra, hysteropathy, metropathy, pneumohydrometra

uterus examination: hysterosalpingography, uterography, uterosalpingography

uterus excision: celiohysterectomy, defundation, fibroidectomy, hysterectomy, hystero-oophorectomy, hysterosalpingectomy, hysterosalpingo-oophorectomy, panhysterectomy, panhysterocolpectomy, panhystero-oophorectomy, panhysterosalpingectomy, panhysterosalpingo-oophorectomy

uterus extrusion: descensus uteri

uterus fixation: exohysteropexy, hysterocystopexy, hysteropexy, trachelectomopexy, uterofixation, uteropexy, ventrohysteropexy, ventrosuspension, ventrovesicofixation

uterus hernia: hysterobubonocele, hysterocele, metrocolpocele, uterocele

uterus incision: abdominohysterotomy, celiohysterotomy, hysterolaparotomy, hysteromyotomy, hysterostomatomy, hysterotomy, hysterotrachelotomy, metrotomy, uterotomy

uterus inflammation: adenomyometritis, adnexitis, endocervicitis, exometritis, hysteritis, lochiometritis, lochometritis, metritis, metroperitonitis, metrophebitis, metrosalpingitis, myometritis, perimetritis, pyometritis, septimetritis

uterus ligament: broad, mesometrium, mesosalpinx

uterus lining: endometrium

uterus membrane: caduca

uterus muscle: myometrium

uterus pain: hysteralgia, metralgia, metrodynia, uteralgia

uterus paralysis: metroparalysis

uterus removal: abdominohysterectomy, hysterectomy, uterectomy

uterus rupture: metrorrhexis

uterus scraping: curettage, endometrectomy

uterus surgery: hysterocleisis, hysterolysis, hysterostomatocleisis, ligamentopexis, metroplasty, uterocystostomy, uteroplasty

uterus suturing: hysterogastrorrhaphy, hysterorrhapy, hysterotrachelorrhaphy

uterus treatment: pessary
uterus tubes: salpingo-, fallopian
tubes
uterus tumors: adenomyoma,
adenomyosis, choriocarcinoma,
chorioepithelioma,
chorionephithelioma, deciduoma,
deciduosarcoma, hysteromyoma,
metrocarcinoma, trophoblastoma
utricle inflammation: utriculitis
uvula: staphylo-
uvula, abnormal: himantosis
uvula, around: peristaphyline
uvula, prolapsed: staphylodialysis,
staphyloptosis, uvulaptosis,
uvuloptosis
uvula fissure: cleft palate,
staphyloschisis
uvula inflammation: staphylitis,
uvulitis
uvula surgery: kiotomy,
staphylectomy, staphyloplasty,
staphylotomy, uvulectomy,
uvulotomy
uvula swelling: staphyledema
uvula tumor: staphyloncus

V

vaccine: attenuated, autogenous,
bacille Calmette-Guerin, brucella,
cholera, duck embryo, influenza,
measles, mumps, paratyphoid,
pertussis, plague, poliomyelitis,
polyvalent, rabies, Rocky Mountain
spotted fever, rubella, Sabin, Salk,
Sauer's, Semple, sensitized,
smallpox, Spencer-Parker,
Staphylococcus, stock,
Streptococcus, tetanus, triple,
typhoid, typhus, univalent, yellow
fever
vaccinelike: vaccinoid
vaccine producing: vaccigenous,
vaccinogenous

vacillate: fluctuate, oscillate, pulsate
vacuole formation: vacuolated
vacuum tube: -tron
vagabond's disease: pediculosis corporis
vagina: cole-, coleo-, colp-, colpo-,
labia majora, labia minora, pronaus
vagina, developed from: vaginogenic
vagina bleeding: colporrhagia,
hematocolpos
vagina changes, in labor: effacement
vagina closing: ankylocolpos, atresia,
colpatresia, gynatresia
vagina dilation: colpectasia, colpeurysis
vagina discharge: fluor albus, gleet,
leukorrhea, lochia
vagina disease: colporrhexis,
hydrocolpos, lochiocolpos,
vaginopathy
vagina dryness: colpoxerosis
vagina examination: colposcopy,
culdocentesis, culdoscopy,
vaginography, vaginoscopy
vagina excision: colpectomy,
vaginectomy
vagina fixation: colpopexy,
vaginapexy, vaginofixation,
vaginopexy
vagina hernia: colpocele, colpocystocele,
enterocele, vaginocele
vagina incision: celiocolpotomy,
coleotomy, colpoceliotomy,
colpocystotomy, colpotomy,
colpostenotomy, episiotomy,
vaginoperineotomy, vaginotomy
vagina infection: vaginomycosis
vagina inflammation: coleocystitis,
colpitis, colpocystitis, encolpitis,
endocolpitis, myocolpitis,
pachycolpismus, pachyvaginitis,
paracolpitis, paravaginitis,
pericolpitis, perivaginitis, vaginitis
vagina pain: colpalgia, colpodynia,
vaginodynia
vagina proplapse: coleoptosis,
colpoptosis
vagina spasm: vaginismus

vagina surgery: colpocleisis,
colpocystoplasty,
colpoperineoplasty,
colpoperineorrhaphy, colpoplasty,
colporrhaphy,
vaginoperineorrhaphy,
vaginoplasty
vagus nerve, act on: vagotropic
vagus nerve, affinity for: vagotropism
vagus nerve hyperirritability:
vagotonia
vagus nerve surgery: vagotomy
vagus nerve inflammation: vagitis
valley fever: coccidioidomycosis
valve: aortic, bicuspid, mitral,
pulmonary, semilunar, tricuspid,
valvula
valve incision: valvotomy, valvulotomy
valve inflammation: valvulitis
vampire: hematophagous
vapor: atmo-, distillation, emanation,
ether, exhalation, steam
variation: deviant, metamorphosis,
mutation
varicose vein examination:
varicography
varicose vein excision: varicotomy
variola-like: varioliform, varioloid
varixlike: cincoid, variciform
vary from normal: poikilo-,
acatastasia
vas deferens excision: gonangiectomy,
vasectomy
vas deferens incision: vasotomy
vas deferens inflammation:
vasovesiculitis
vas deferens puncture: vasopuncture
vas deferens surgery:
vasoepididymostomy, vaso-
orchidostomy, vasosection,
vasostomy, vasovasostomy
vasomotor nerve disease:
angioneuropathy, vasoneurosis
vasomotor nerve paralysis: vasoparesis
vasopressors: dopamine, ephedrine,
epinephrine, mephentermine,
metaraminol, methoxamine,
norepinephrine, phenylephrine

vegetative nervous system: autonomic
nervous system
vein: phleb-, phlebo-, veno-, -venous,
vena, venule
vein, bleeding from: phleborrhagia
vein, science of: phlebology
vein aneurysm: phlebangioma
vein calculus: phlebolith
vein compression: phlebostasis
vein contraction: venospasm
vein dilation: phlebectasia, phlebismus,
varicosity, varix
vein diseases: hemorrhoids,
phlebocholosis, phlebothrombosis,
varicose
vein displacement: phlebectopia
vein examination: phlebography,
venography
vein excision: phlebectomy,
varicotomy, venectomy
vein hardening: phlebosclerosis,
venosclerosis
vein incision: phlebotomy, venesection,
venisection, venotomy
vein inflammation: periphlebitis,
peripylephlebitis, phlebitis,
thrombophlebitis, varicophlebitis
veinlike: phleboid
vein obstruction: phlebemphraxis
vein puncture: venipuncture
vein rupture: phleborrhexis
veins, major: portal, pulmonary, vena
cava
vein surgery: Babcock's operation,
phleboplasty, venovenostomy
vein suturing: phleborrhaphy,
venisuture
vena cava inflammation: cavitis,
celophlebitis
venereal disease, fear of:
cypridophobia, venereophobia
venereal disease, study of: cypridology,
venereology
venereal diseases: acquired immune
deficiency syndrome, balanitis
gangrenosa, chancroid, condyloma
acuminatum, Frei's disease,
gonorrhea, granuloma inguinale,
herpesvirus, lymphogranuloma

venereum, Nicolas-Favre disease,
sexually transmitted diseases,
syphilis
venereal disease specialist:
venereologist
venereal sore: chancre
venereal warts: condyloma, verruca
acuminata
venom: lethal, poison, toxin, virulent
venom, against: antitoxin, antivenin
venom, inactivated: anavenin
venous hum: bruit de diable
ventilation: catharsis, respiration
ventral: ventri-, ventro-, abneural
ventricle: ventriculo-, camera
vertebra: spondyl-, spondylo-,
vertebro-, atlas, axis, cervical,
thoracic, lumbar, sacral, coccygeal
vertebra diseases: ankylosing
spondylitis, platyspondylisis, Pott's
disease, spondylarthritis,
spondylarthrocace, spondylocace,
spondylopathy, tuberculosis
vertebra disintegration: spondylolysis
vertebra dislocation:
spondylexarthrosis,
spondylolisthesis
vertebra excision: laminectomy,
transversectomy, vertebrectomy
vertebra fissure: rhachischisis,
schistorrhachis, spina bifida,
spondyloschisis
vertebra fusion: spondylosis,
spondylosyndesis
vertebra inflammation: perispondylitis,
spondylarthritis, rachitis,
spondylitis
vertebral column: rachi-, rachio-,
backbone, rachis, spinal column
vertebral column, fluid in: rachiochysis
vertebral column abnormality:
rachiopagus
vertebral column curvature: crytosis,
kyphorrachitis, kyphoscoliosis,
kyphosis, kyrtorrhachic,
lordoscoliosis, lordosis,
rachiocampsis, rachioscoliosis,
scoliosis, trachelokyphosis

**vertebral column curvature
measurement:** rachigraphy,
rachiometry, scoliosiometry,
scoliosometry
vertebral column surgery: rachiotomy,
spondylotomy
vertebral column treatment:
chiropractic, chymopapain,
rachilysis, spondylotherapy,
traction
vertebral process, accessory:
anapophysis
vertebra pain: spinalgia, spondylalgia,
spondylodynia
vertigo therapy: antidinic, belladonna,
dimenhydrinate,
diphenhydramine, diphenidol,
hyoscyamine, meclizine,
promethazine, scopolamine
verumontanum: colliculus
verumontanum excision: colliculectomy
verumontanum inflammation:
colliculitis, verumontanitis
vesicle excision: vesiculectomy
vesicle formation: vesiculation
vesicle incision: vesiculotomy
vesicle inflammation: vesiculitis
vesicle-shaped: vesiculiform
vessel: angei-, angi-, angio-, vaso-,
ampule, artery, beaker, flask, phial,
test tube, vein, vial
vessel diameter: caliber
vessel pain: vasalgia
vessels, new: vasifactive, vasofactive,
vasoformative
vibration: fremitus, oscillation,
palpitation, pulsation, resonance
vibration, lack of sensation:
apallesthesia, pallanesthesia
vibration, nonperception of:
hypopallesthesia
vibration sensation: pallesthesia,
seismesthesia
vibration therapy: seismotherapy,
sismotherapy, vibromassage
view: -scope

viewer: endoscope, fiberscope, observerscope

villus inflammation: villositis

vinegar: acet-

violet blindness: anianthinopsy, ianthinopsia

virginity loss: defloration

virus, bacterial: bacteriophage, phage

virus, study of: virology

virus destroying: viricidal, virucidal

virus disease: Argentine hemorrhagic fever, Bolivian hemorrhagic fever, Borna, Bornhalm, Bwamba fever, Burkitt's lymphoma, chickenpox, Colorado tick fever, common cold, cowpox, coxsackievirus, Crimean-Congo hemorrhagic fever, cytomegalovirus, dengue, encephalitis, encephalomyelitis, epidemic keratoconjunctivitis, epidemic pleurodynia, equine encephalitis, hemorrhagic fever, hepatitis, herpangina, herpes, infectious bronchitis, influenza, kuru, Lassa fever, leukemia, leukoencephalopathy, Marburg disease, measles, mumps, mononucleosis, Newcastle, panencephalitis, pneumonia. poliomyelitis, rabies, Rift Valley fever, St. Louis encephalitis, shingles, smallpox, varicella, variola, yellow fever

viruses: adenovirus, arbovirus, amphotrophic, arenavirus, attenuated, bunyavirus, California, coronavirus, echovirus, Epstein-Barr, hepatitis, herpesvirus, myxovirus, oncornavirus, orphan, papovavirus, paramyxovirus, picornavirus, poliovirus, poxvirus. reovirus, rhinovirus, rotavirus, slow, togavirus

virus in blood: viremia, virusemia

virus in urine: viruria

virus particle: virion

virus therapy: acyclovir, amantadine, antiviral, aranotin, arildone, avridine, cytarabine, edoxudine, enviradene, famotine, floxuridine, fosarilate, foscarnet, fosfonet, idoxuridine, interferon, kethoxal, memotine, methisazone, ribavirin, rimantadine, somantadine, statolon, steffimycin, tilorone, trifluridine, vidarabine, viroxime, zinviroxime

visage: physiognomy

viscera: viscero-, splanchnic
    See also abdomen, intestine

viscera diseases: splanchanectopia, splanchnodiastasis, splanchnopathy

viscera examination: splanchnoscopy

viscera excision: splanchnicectomy

viscera hardening: splanchnosclerosis

viscera inflammation: perisplanchnitis, perivisceritis

viscera prolapse: splanchnoptosia, visceroptosis

viscera sensation: splanchesthetia

viscera surgery: devisceration, evisceration, splanchnicotomy, splanchnotomy

visible: patent, phanic

vision: opto-, eye, eyesight, oculus, sight

vision, abnormal: anorthopia, aphose, cyanopsia, dysmegalopsia, dysmetropsia, dysopia, hemianopsia, myopia, parablepsia, presbyopia, pseudoblepsia, pseudopsia, strabismus, triplopia

vision, acute: oxyblepsia, oxyopia

vision, blurred: halation, hemeralopia

vision, color: retinal cone

vision, dim: amblyopia, asthenopia, caligo, nephelopia

vision, double: ambiopia, amphodipolpia, amphoterodipolpia, dipolpia, monodiplopia

vision, normal: emmetropia, stereopsis

vision, poor at night: nyctalopia, nyctamblyopia, nyctotyphlosis

vision, single: haplopia
vision, unequal: anisopia, heteropsia
vision correction: orthoptics
vision diseases: diplopia, Leber's
congenital amaurosis, monoblepsia,
paropsic, peripheriphose,
peripherophose, polyopia,
psychanopsia, psychic blindness,
scieropia, tunnel vision
vision measurement: campimetry
vision sensitivity: optesthesia
visual purple: rhodopsin
vitality, depleted: asthenia
vitality loss: devitalization
vital processes, restored: anabiosis
vital signs: body temperature, pulse
rate, respiration rate; blood
pressure
vitamin, study of: vitaminology
vitamin A: retinol
vitamin A deficiency: nyctalophia,
xerophthalmia
vitamin A excess: carotenemia
vitamin B complex: biotin, choline,
cobalamine, cyanocobalamin, folic
acid, niacin, nicotinamide, nicotinic
acid, pantothenic acid, para-
aminobenzoic acid, pyridoxamine,
pyridoxine, riboflavin, thiamine
vitamin B complex deficiency:
ariboflavinosis, berberi, cheilosis,
pellagra, macrocytic anemia,
pernicious anemia
vitamin C: ascorbic acid
vitamin C deficiency: Barlow's disease
infantile scurvy, scurvy
vitamin C in blood, excessive:
ascorbemia
vitamin C in urine, excessive:
ascorburia
vitamin D: calciferol, cholecalciferol,
ergocalciferol, ergosterol, viosterol
vitamin D deficiency: rickets
vitamin deficiency: avitaminosis,
hypovitaminosis
vitamin E: tocopherol

vitamin H: biotin
vitamin K: menadione, phytonadione
vitamin-like: vitamoid
vitamin P: bioflavonoid
vitamins, excessive: hypervitaminosis,
supervitaminosis
vitiligo therapy: trioxsalen
vitreous body surgery: hyalonyxis
vitreous humor inflammation: hyalitis,
hyaloiditis, vitreocapsulitis
vocal cord excision: chordectomy
vocal cord inflammation: chorditis,
myochorditis
voice: phon-, phono-, articulation,
phonal, vox
voice, clear: lamprophonia
voice, fear of one's: phonophobia
voice, impaired: dysphonia
voice, masculine, in woman:
androglossia
voice, nasal: mycterophonia,
rhinolalia, rhinophonia
voice, normal: euphonia
voice, rough: trachyphonia
voice, shrill: oxyphonia
voice, study of: phoniatrics
voice, weak: hypophonia, leptophonia,
phonasthenia
voice box: larynx
voice change: heterophonia
voice disorder: olophonia, paraphonia
voice loss: aphonia, apsithyria, mute,
nyctaphonia, nyctophonia
voice producing: glottis, vocal cords
voices: hallucinations
void: defecation, discharge, ejection,
emission, evacuation, micturition,
urination
voids, fear of: cenophobia, kenophobia
volatile: evaporating, unstable,
vaporizing
vomiting: antiperistalsis, emesis
vomiting, excessive: anacatharsis,
hyperemesis
vomiting, fear of: emetophobia
vomiting, inducing: anacathartic,
emetic, emetine, vomitory

vomiting, preventive: antemetic,
  antiemetic
vomiting attempt: retch, vomiturition
vomiting blood: hematemesis
vomiting feces: copremesis
voracious: bulimia, polyphagia
voyeurism: scopophilia
vulnerable: susceptible
vulva disease: vulvopathy
vulva excision: vulvectomy
vulva glands: Bartholin's, vulvovaginal
vulva incision: episiotomy
vulva inflammation: vulvovaginitis
vulva slit narrowing: episiostenosis
vulva surgery: episioclisia,
  episioperineoplasty, episioplasty
vulva suturing: episioperineorrhaphy,
  episiorrhaphy

W

wakefulness: consciousness, insomnia,
  pervigilium, sleeplessness, vigil
walk: ambulation, gait
walk, inability to: abasia
walk altered: festination, helicopodia,
  scissor, spastic, tabetic waddling
walk backward, involuntary:
  opisthoporeia, retropulsion
walking: ambulant, orthograde
walking ability: -basia
walking, fear of: basiphobia,
  basophobia, stasibasiphobia
walking difficulty: abasia, dysbasia
walk on hands and feet: pronograde
walk on sole of foot: plantigrade
wall: dissipiment, membrane, paries,
  septate, septulum, septum
walleye: divergent strabismus
wan: anemic, ashen, pale, pallor
wandering: aberrant, floating,
  migratory, peripatetic
wandering impulse: drapetomania,
  dromomania
wanderlust: drapetomania,
  dromomania, ecdemomania

wane: abate, degenerate, deteriorate,
  subside
warm: fever, tepid
warm blooded: hemathermous,
  homoiothermic, homothermic
warmth producing: calefacient
warning: indication, sign, symptom
wart: condyloma, sycoma, thymion,
  verruca
wartlike: verruciform, verrucose
wash: disinfect, douche, flush, irrigate,
  lavage, retrojection
washing, excessive: ablutomania
waste matter: biodetritus, detritus,
  egesta, emunctory, feces, menses,
  phytodetritus, stool, sweat, tartar,
  urine, zoodetritus
waste removal: depurant
wasting: atrophy, cachexia,
  colliquation, decay, degeneration,
  deterioration, dystrophy,
  emaciation, macies, marasmus,
  metatrophia, myatrophy,
  panatrophy, pedatrophy, phthisis,
  symptosis, syntexis, tabes
wasting of leg calves: acnemia
water: hydr-, hydro-, aqua, aqueus,
  saliva, sweat, tears, urine
water, excess in blood: hydremia
water, fear of: hydrophobia,
  potamophobia
water, lack of: anhydrous
water, make: micturition, urination
water, reaction with: hydrolysis
water, science of: hydrology
waterbrash: heartburn, pyrosis
water compound: hydrate
water cure: hydrotherapy
water deficiency: anhydrous,
  dehydration, hydropenia,
  hydropericardium
water hernia: hydrocephalocele
water in a sac: blister, hydrocele
water in fallopian tube:
  hydroparasalpinx
water in parotid gland: hydroparotitis

water in spinal canal: hydromyelocele
water in spinal cord: hydromyelia
water in umbilicus: hydromphalus
water in uterus: hydrometra,
    hydrophysometra
water loss: dehydration, plasmolysis
water of eye: aqueous humor
water on the brain: hydrencephalus,
    hydrocephalus, hydroencephalus
water on the knee: hydrarthrosis
water pill: diuretic
water removal: dehydration
water retention: edema, hydropexis,
    hydrophilism
waters: amniotic fluid
water treatment: aquapuncture,
    aspersion, dipsotherapy,
    hydriatrics, hydropathy,
    hydrosudotherapy, hydrotherapy
watery mixture: slurry
wavelike motion: oscillation,
    undulation
waves: peristalsis
wavy: sinuous, undulate
wax: cer-, cera-, cerumen
weak: amyous, debilitated, flaccid,
    hyposthenic, inanition, infirm,
    invalid, senile, valetudinarian
weaken: reduce
weakened: attenuated
weakness: adynamia, amyosthenia,
    asthenia, atonia, atrophy, cachexia,
    catheresis, debility, disability,
    enervation, malaise, myasthenia,
    neurasthenia, panasthenia
weak reflexes: hyporeflexia
weaning: ablactation, delactation
wear away: abrasion, attrition,
    degenerate, detrition, excoriation,
    slough
weariness: apocammosis, fatigue,
    lethargy
web-fingered: symphalangism,
    syndactyly
weblike: arachnoid, tela, textiform
web-toed: symphalangism, syndactyly

wedge: cuneo-, spheno-
wedged in: impacted
weed: cannabis
weeping: lacrimation
weight: bar-, baro-, ponderal
weight perception: barognosis
weight perception, lack of:
    abarognosis, baragnosis
well: eu-
wen: pilar cyst, sebaceous cyst,
    steatoma
wet: hygro-
wet dream: nocturnal emission
wheal: pomphus, urtica, whelk
wheat allergy: celiac disease
wheeze: rhoncus
whipping: flagellation
whipworm: Trichuris
whirlbone: patella
whirlpool: vortex
whiskey face: acne rosacea
whisper: susurrus
whistle: sibilant, syrigmophonia
white: alb-, alba-, leuk-, leuko-,
    anemia, pallor
white blood cells: basophil, B-cell,
    eosinophil, granulocyte, leukocyte,
    lymphocyte, macrophage,
    microphage, monoblast, monocyte,
    neutrophil, phagocyte,
    polymorphonuclear leukocyte, T-
    cell
white blood cells, decreased:
    agranulocytosis, anisohypocytosis,
    granulocytopenia, hypoeosinophilia,
    hypolymphemia, hyponeocytosis,
    leukocytopenia, leukopenia,
    neutropenia
white blood cells, destruction:
    leukocytolysis, leukolysis, leukotoxia
white blood cells, formation:
    leukocytopoiesis, leukopoiesis
white blood cells, immature: -blast,
    leukoblast, leukocytoblast,
    myeloblast, myeloplast,
    promyelocyte, skeocytosis

white blood cells, increased:
anisohypercytosis,
hyperarthocytosis, hypercytosis,
hyperleukocytosis, hyperneocytosis,
leukemia, leukocytopenia,
leukocytosis, leukopenia,
neutropenia, normoorthocytosis,
pleocytosis

white blood cells in urine: leukocyturia

white hair: achromotrichia, canities,
leukotricia, poliosis

whitehead: milium

white leg: phlebitis, phlegmasia alba
dolens

white mouth: cancidiasis, candidosis,
moniliasis

white of eye: conjunctiva, sclera

white spots: leukokeratosis, leukoma,
leukoplakia, leukoplasia

whitlow: felon, panaris, paronychia

whole: hol-, holo-, pant-, panto-

wholesome: roborant, salubrious

whooping cough: pertussis

whorl: convoluted, helix, vortex

wide: eury-, platy-

widow's hump: kyphosis

will: -bulia, bulesis, conation

will power, abnormal: abulia,
hypobulia, parabulia

will power, excessive: hyperbulia

wind: anemo-, borborygmus,
crepitation, flatus

wind, away: anemotropism

wind, fear of: anemophobia

wind, toward: anemotropism

winding: anfractuous, convoluted,
flexuous, sinuous, tortuous

winding sheet: shroud

windpipe: trachea

windpipe covering: epiglottis

wing: pinna

winglike: ala

wing-shaped: alate, aliform, pterygoid

wink: nictitate, palpebrate

wipe: swab

wisdom tooth: dens serotinus, third
molar

wishbone: furcula

with: co-, con-, sym-

withdrawal: abduction, coitus
interruptus, retraction,
retrogression

wither: desiccate, shrivel, wrinkle

withhold: restraint

within: end-, endo-, ent-, ento-, eso-,
intra-, intro-, internal

without: a-, an-, ecto-, ex-, exo-,
extra-, extro-, external

without echoes: anechoic

withstand: resistance

woman: gyn-, gyne-, gyneco-, gyno-,
female

woman, bearded: Achard-Thiers
syndrome

woman, male characteristics:
virilescence

woman, old: anility

womanhater: gynephobe, misogynist

womanly: gynecoid

womb: uterus

women's diseases: gynecology,
gynecopathy

women's diseases, treatment of:
gyniatrics

wood: xylo-

wood alcohol: methanol

word blindness: alexia, aphasia,
aphemesthesia, dyslexia

word deafness: auditory amnesia,
kophemia, logokophosis

word repetition: autoecholalia,
echolalia

words: logo-
See also speech

words, misunderstanding: sensory
aphasia

words, misuse: paramnesia,
paraphasia, paraphemia

work: ergo-, pono-, ergonomics

work, dread of: aphilopony

workaholic: ergasiomania

work therapy: ergotherapy

work together: synergism

worm destroyer: vermicide
worm diseases: ancylostomicus, anisakiniasis, ascariasis, enterobiasis, filiariasis, helminthiasis, hookworm, onchocerciasis, strongyloidiasis, trichinosis, trichuriasis
wormlike: helminthoid, lumbrical, sinuous, tortuous, vermicular, vermiform
worms: Ascaris, Echinococcus, Fasciola, Filaria, fluke, helminth, Hymenolepis, Necator, Nematode, Oesophagostomum, Onchocerca, Opisthorchis, Paragonimus, pinworm, seatworm, Termatoda, Trichinella, Trichuris, vermis
worms, drug for: anthelmintic
worms, fear of: helminthophobia, vermiphobia
worms, study of: helminthology, nematology
worms, treatment: helminthagogue, helminthicide, vermicide, vermifuge
worms, tumor from: helminthoma
worms, vomiting: helminthemesis
wormwood: absinthium
worsening: degeneration, deterioration, exacerbation, progression, retrogression
wound: abrasion, contusion, injury, laceration, lesion, puncture, trauma, vulnerate, vulnus
wound, exclusion of air: anaeroplasty
wound, science of: traumatology
wound healing preventive: antiplastic
wound retraction: anastole
wound trimming: revivification, vivification
wrap: encapsulate, pack
wrench: sprain, strain, twist
wrinkle: crevice, corrugate, furrow, line, ridge, rugose
wrinkle removal: rhitidectomy, rhytidectomy, rhytidoplasty

wrist: carpus
wrist bones: scaphoid, lunate, triangular, pisiform, trapezium, trapezoid, capitate, hamate
wrist drop: carpoptosis
wrist joint: radiocarpal articulation
wrist surgery: metacarpectomy
write, inability to: agraphia, dysgraphia
write, with both hands: ambidextrous
write nonsense: graphorrhea
write on skin: graphesthesia
writer's cramp: cheirospasm, dysgraphia, graphospasm
writing analysis: graphology
writing disorder: agitographia, agraphia, anorthography, dysantigraphia, heterography, logagraphia, palingraphia, paragraphia, pseudographia
written order: prescription
wrong: mis-
wryneck: torticollis

X

xanthine in urine, excessive: xanthinuria, xanthiuria, xanthuria
xiphoid process inflammation: xiphoiditis
xiphoid process pain: xiphodynia
x-ray: computed tomography, radiograph, roentgenogram, roentgenography, xeroradiography
x-shaped: decussation

Y

yawning: oscedo, oscitation, pandiculation, scordinema
yaws: bouba, bubas, frambesia, parangi, patek, pian
yaws lesion: frambesioma
yeast: fermentum, fungus

yellow: flav-, flavo-, xanth-, xantho-,
    subflavous, xanthelasma, xanthic,
    xanthochromic
yellow bile: humor
yellow blindness: axanthopsia
yellow fever transmitter: Aedes
    aegypti
yellow marrow: bone marrow
yellow pigment: lutein
yellow pigment in blood: carotenemia,
    xanthemia
yellow skin: icterus, jaundice,
    xanthochromia
yield: reproduce
yielding: ductile, elastic, flaccid,
    flexible, resilient
yolk: zyg-, zygo-, vitelline
yolk, absent: alecithal
yolk, diminished: oligolecithal

yolk membrane: vitelline membrane
young: adolescent, child, ephebic,
    juvenile, pubescent
young, study of: ephebiatrics
youthful looking: agerasia
y-shaped: ypsiliform

Z

zenith: apex, crown, head, vertex
zigzag: anfractuous, sinuous
zinclike: zincoid
zinc poisoning: zincalism
zone: area, region, section, zona,
    zonula, zonule
zone, away from: zonifugal
zone, toward: zonipetal